I0094530

Auxiliaries in Primary Health Care
An Annotated Bibliography

Edited by Dr Katherine Elliott
Assistant Director of the Ciba Foundation
Honorary Director of AHRTAG

Compiled by the Appropriate Health Resources &
Technologies Action Group (AHRTAG)

Practical
ACTION
PUBLISHING

Practical Action Publishing Ltd
27a Albert Street, Rugby, CV21 2SG, Warwickshire, UK
www.practicalactionpublishing.org

© Intermediate Technology Publications 1979

First published 1979
Transferred to digital printing 2008

ISBN 978 0 903031 58 5

All rights reserved. No part of this publication may be reprinted or reproduced or utilized in any form or by any electronic, mechanical, or other means, now known or hereafter invented, including photocopying and recording, or in any information storage or retrieval system, without the written permission of the publishers.

A catalogue record for this book is available from the British Library.

The contributors have asserted their rights under the Copyright Designs and Patents Act 1988 to be identified as authors of their respective contributions.

Since 1974, Practical Action Publishing has published and disseminated books and information in support of international development work throughout the world. Practical Action Publishing is a trading name of Practical Action Publishing Ltd (Company Reg. No. 1159018), the wholly owned publishing company of Practical Action. Practical Action Publishing trades only in support of its parent charity objectives and any profits are covenanted back to Practical Action (Charity Reg. No. 247257, Group VAT Registration No. 880 9924 76).

Acknowledgments

This publication was made possible by a generous grant from the Ministry of Overseas Development.
The Intermediate Technology Development Group greatly acknowledges the Ministry's assistance.

We thank our many friends who have contributed to our collection of manuals and other documents.
We thank the World Health Organization, the Ministry of Overseas Development of the United Kingdom, and the Leverhulme Trust through the International Hospital Federation for making it possible to bring the Appropriate Health Resources and Technologies Action Group into being. We very much appreciate the personal encouragement given to us by the Director-General of WHO, Dr Halfdan Mahler, in his generous foreword to this bibliography.

I myself particularly want to thank my AHRTAG colleagues who have borne the brunt of the work involved in putting the bibliography together: Arna Blum, Maureen Gadd, Cathy Last, Chris Lomax and especially Mavis Solomon and Sunil Mehra.

K.E.

Contents

Foreword by Dr Halfdan Mahler, Director-General, WHO   iv

Introduction   v

Section 1—Education and Training of Auxiliaries in   1
       Primary Health Care

Section 2—Auxiliaries and Community Health and   33
       Development

Appendix 1—Geographical Index   84

Appendix 2—Subject Index   86

Appendix 3—Useful Addresses   91

Appendix 4—Journals referred to in the Bibliography   113

Appendix 5—Publishers referred to in the Bibliography   117

Foreword

This is indeed a useful venture. Since the first edition was published the Member States of the World Health Organization have committed themselves to the decisive socio-economic task of providing health for all by the year 2000. This cannot be achieved through the conventional health service development of the past few decades. Primary health care is a new concept which demands action at the social periphery, where the old order rarely penetrated. The health auxiliary will play a vital role in this re-orientation of health services towards increased social relevance.

This new bibliography will provide a valuable reference for all those concerned with the training and supervision of health auxiliaries. The better their task in primary health care is understood, the better will they be prepared for their work.

It is a pleasure to preface this edition with the good wishes of the World Health Organization for its success.

H. Mahler, M.D.
Director General
World Health Organization

Introduction

Primary health care begins with human beings, families, homes and communities and cannot be separated out from general social and economic improvement. Everyone must have access to primary health care, find its form and its costs acceptable, and be willing to participate appropriately. To meet complex health needs, referral routes to specialist medical services must be provided and safe-guarded. Auxiliary workers can nevertheless carry most of the primary health care burden because experience has shown that primary health care services work most satisfactorily when they make use of local people, who remain part of the communities they serve but who have been given the right kind of technical and social training to enable them to respond effectively to local needs. They then become an invaluable resource for the new style of health services which are required to meet the target set by the World Health Organization of health for all by the year 2000.

In most countries now health services are being reshaped with greater flexibility in mind. New ways are being sought and found to train and to integrate increasing numbers of auxiliary health workers in systems which inevitably vary by country and by community according to the needs to be met and the human and material resources available for this purpose. Much more is being recorded about the different approaches being tried and attempts have been made to evaluate some of them. This revised version of a previous annotated bibliography, *The Training of Auxiliaries in Health Care* (Intermediate Technology Publications, 1975), is intended to promote the greater exchange of know-how, of useful teaching materials and background information, and to encourage wider experimentation. Knowledge needs to be shared in a field where so much still remains to be done. This small book sets out what the Appropriate Health Resources and Technologies Action Group Ltd (AHRTAG) is aware of as being of potential use to anyone interested in health auxiliaries and in primary health care.

The Appropriate Health Resources and Technologies Action Group Ltd (AHRTAG) is a non-profit organization established in 1977, with the approval and encouragement of the late Dr E. F. Schumacher, to replace the Rural Health Panel of the Intermediate Technology Development Group (ITDG). AHRTAG maintains close links with ITDG and was designated an official WHO Collaborating Centre early in 1978. AHRTAG's purpose is to promote the appropriate and effective delivery of primary health care in all parts of the world. It acts as a clearing-house for information about useful alternatives to high cost, high technology, hospital-based medical practice. It encourages innovation, offers liaison and catalytic services, and can recommend technical consultants. It maintains and is expanding a diverse international network of personal contacts, all of whom have experience and expertise to offer in connection with health and community development.

Katherine Elliott

Education and Training of Auxiliaries in Primary Health Care

1 **African Medical and Research Foundation,** *Afya: A Journal for Medical and Health Workers.* African Medical and Research Foundation, Nairobi. This monthly publication features articles on diagnostic and treatment procedures for lower and middle level health workers. Articles on topics such as nutrition, hygiene, integrated health projects, and health centres are written in simple terms with appropriate illustrations. Of interest to medical and health workers in developing countries.

2 **Alaska, Department of Health and Welfare,** *Midwifery Teaching Guide for Public Health Nurses.* Department of Health and Welfare, Juneau, Alaska, 1966, 39 pp. This guide is written for nurse-midwives to assist in the instruction of traditional village midwives and local mothers in hygienic midwifery practices. It is divided into three parts, and deals with the planning of classes, course content, and teaching schedules. It also gives a list of teaching aids. Useful source material for teachers of auxiliaries.

3 **Alaska, U.S. Public Health Service,** *Alaska Community Health Aide Training Manual.* U.S. Public Health Service, 1973, 454 pp. This manual aims to provide general information about the Alaska Community Health Aide Training Programme for persons within and outside Alaska Area Health Service. A useful guide for health aides.

4 **All Africa Leprosy and Rehabilitation Training Centre (ALERT),** *Rural Area Supervisors Course: Jan–May 1971 Lecture Notes.* ALERT, Addis Ababa, (no date), 170 pp. These notes are designed to supplement the WHO Guide to Leprosy Control and ALERT's Simple Guide to Leprosy. They cover basic science, clinical methods, rehabilitation, and leprosy control programmes. Discussions on clinics, epidemiology, case finding, and evaluation procedures are included. Duties and training of health workers are also discussed.

5 **All Africa Leprosy and Rehabilitation Training Centre (ALERT),** *Health Education Kit*

1

for Teachers. ALERT, Addis Ababa, 1974, 16 pp. This useful kit is designed to inform teachers in Ethiopia of modern views on leprosy which can be taught in schools. It emphasizes the importance of early treatment, and is illustrated with exercises to test readers' comprehension.

6   **All Africa Leprosy and Rehabilitation Training Centre (ALERT),** *A Footwear Manual for Leprosy Control Programmes (Part 1).* Edited by Neville, P. Jane, ALERT, Addis Ababa, 1977, 45 pp. This manual is based on many decades of experience with leprosy patients in Africa. The contributors are still actively involved in the care of patients and this is the first attempt to document the medical, technical and managerial aspects of providing footwear, and other necessary appliances for rehabilitating them. The causes and treatment of wounds on the feet are dealt with in detail. A good example of an integrative, entrepreneurial approach.

7   **All Africa Leprosy and Rehabilitation Training Centre (ALERT),** *A Footwear Manual for Leprosy Control Programmes (Part 2).* Edited by Neville, P. Jane, ALERT, Addis Ababa, 1977, 118 pp. Part 2 of this manual deals with basic procedures such as the tools required, measuring, marking and cutting, joining, finishing and fitting of footwear for leprosy patients. Section III gives the construction details of different footwear, such as the simple sandal, the tyre sandal, modified canvas boot, etc., and the foot drop brace, the fixed ankle brace walker, the kneeling prosthesis and ulcer healing leg, crutches. The appendices include basic tools for a small workshop, a list of suppliers, and tools and materials for a rural clinic.

8   **Anderson, B. G.,** *Obstetrics for the Nurse.* Delmar Publications, New York, 1972, 176 pp. Although written for American nurses or midwives, this book, which is in simple language, could be useful for teachers of auxiliaries, and for auxiliaries when teaching mothers. It covers conception, the growth of the foetus, and has practical notes on managing prenatal, parturition and postpartum care, but gives details of hospital delivery procedures only. A sample clinical record and an index are included.

9   **Arnhold, Rainer,** *The Arm Circumference as a Public Health Index of Protein-Calorie Malnutrition of Early Childhood.* Journal of Tropical Paediatrics (London), Vol. 15, No. 4, Dec. 1969, Reprint available from Institute of Child Health, London, 5 pp. This leaflet describes the principle and application of the 'Quacstick', which uses arm-circumference-for-height of a child as a simple diagnosis of protein-calorie malnutrition in young children. The 'Quacstick'

is very useful in assessing nutritional standards in communities and for screening children, and is a valuable tool to teach health workers about child nutrition.

10 Assar, M., *Guide to Sanitation in Natural Disasters.* WHO, Geneva, 1971, 143 pp. The contents, which include pre-disaster and post-disaster measures such as medical services, sanitation, and sanitary engineering, emphasize the need for coordination of government and private efforts. Annexes include a list of equipment and supplies, a summary of sanitary requirements, and instructions for disinfection of water supplies. These are measures which could be useful even during normal situations in developing countries.

11 Backs, M. and Bicknell, W. J., *Medical Assistant: A Compendium.* Office of Health Affairs, Office of Economic Opportunity, San Francisco, 1970, 459 pp. A project to train native Alaskans as middle level auxiliaries was undertaken by the Office of Economic Opportunity. To gather background material for suitable curriculum and lesson plans, the project administrators contacted officers of similar programmes throughout the world. The results of their investigations have been assembled in this document. Curricula from civilian and military courses are outlined, and resource personnel

are cited. A catalogue of related materials is included.

12 Biddulph, John, *Child Health for Health Extension Officers.* Port Moresby General Hospital, Boroko, Papua New Guinea, 1973, 210 pp. This book is intended for use as a training and reference manual for Health Extension Officers in rural Papua New Guinea. Although it emphasizes the care and treatment of diseases likely to be found in children, chapters on preventive medicine, food and nutrition, maternal and child health, family planning, and health education are included. There are numerous illustrations, an index, and a table of drug dosages for children.

13 Biddulph, John, *Standardized Management of Diarrhoea in Young Children.* Tropical Doctor (London), Vol. 2, 1972, pp. 114–117. This article describes a simple standardized treatment and diagnosis, which can be performed by adequately trained auxiliary staff. It covers intravenous rehydration, breastfeeding, and administration of oral fluids. Very useful article for all those working in community health.

14 Bomgaars, M. and Bajracharya, B., *Symptom-treatment Manual.* Shanta Bhawan Hospital, Kathmandu, 1974, 42 pp. This manual contains brief descriptions of symptoms, possible complications, and simple treatments suitable for use by para-professional health staff. It is indexed, with separate sub-sections devoted to the recognition and treatment of eye, ear, nose and throat infections, common diseases, women's conditions, complications which may affect the new born, family planning, and immunization. It also includes a detailed list of basic drugs with recommended dosages for children and adults.

15 **Bowler, D. P.,** *Child Health Manual for Community Nurses.* WHO, in conjunction with Department of Health, Papua New Guinea, available from REMAHA, 1973, 159 pp. This manual covers most aspects of child health care, including illnesses of the newborn, infectious diseases, some common childhood diseases, etc. There is also a section on maternal health. Basic nursing knowledge is assumed. Symptoms, diagnosis, treatment, and drugs are dealt with in the relevant sections. Very useful, and applicable to auxiliaries in other regions. Also available in French (see entry 137) and a Portuguese version is in preparation.

16 **British Red Cross Society,** *ABC of First Aid.* British Red Cross Society, London, 1968, 35 pp. Step by step instructions for first-aid are provided in this brief, simple and comprehensive booklet. It explains treatment for such emergencies as

abdominal, chest, and eye injuries, for childbirth and miscarriage, and for fractures, poisoning, nosebleeds, heart attack, fainting, animal and insect bites, burns, scalds, etc. Included are lists of first-aid materials for a home kit.

17 **British Red Cross Society,** *Practical First Aid.* British Red Cross Society, London, 1972, 94 pp. This manual briefly explains that first-aid is emergency treatment given until proper medical attention can be obtained. It describes the normal functions of the body and explains the causes and evidence of malfunction. Simple treatment is outlined for such conditions as burns, fractures, snake bites and insect stings. Shock and hysteria are also discussed. Most of the information is relevant for developing countries. Methods of making stretchers and splints from available materials are illustrated.

18 **British Red Cross Society,** *Nursing Junior Manual and Practical Nursing.* British Red Cross Society, London, 1977, 64 pp., supplement 10 pp. This simply written material could be universally applicable as it covers basic principles for the care of sick and disabled patients. It includes medication, treatment of inflammation, care of wounds, communicable diseases, and the care of handicapped children and the elderly. Appendices contain a summary of infectious diseases

4

and syllabi for two levels of nursing auxiliaries.

19 **Bryceson, A. and Pfaltzgraff, R. E.**, *Leprosy for Students of Medicine.* Churchill Livingstone, Edinburgh, 1973, 152 pp. Chapters of this book include symptoms and signs, diagnosis, treatment, and immunology of leprosy. References and further reading lists are given at the end of each chapter. It is excellent value and, although written for medical students, should be useful for higher levels of auxiliary health personnel, and as a source book for people planning training courses or writing manuals for auxiliaries.

20 **Burgess, H. J. L.**, *Protein Calorie Malnutrition in Children.* Ross Institute, London, 1970, 31 pp. This deals in detail with the description and diagnosis, causes, prevention, and treatment of mild and severe cases of malnutrition. Preventive measures include improved agricultural practices, local support of nutrition and health education, and an improvement in health services. Appendices provide dietary details. A useful booklet.

21 **Busvine, J. R.**, *The Housefly and its Control.* Ross Institute, London, 1970, 27 pp. Control of the housefly, a great threat to the health of people throughout the world, is this pamphlet's aim. Insecticides and curative methods cannot substitute for proper sanitation, and the most efficient and practical method is to check the breeding of flies by adequate sanitary disposal of human and animal excreta and garbage. All possible methods of controlling the spread of the housefly are listed.

22 **Byrne, M. and Bennett, F. J.**, *Community Nursing in Developing Countries, a Manual for the Auxiliary Public Health Nurse.* Oxford University Press, London/Nairobi, 1973, 208 pp. Written from experience in Uganda, this manual gives practical advice for effective home visiting and public health nursing, health education, and improvement of community health. It has sections on communicable diseases, the care of the young child, home economics, and the learning process, and should be useful for high level auxiliaries and their training in developing countries. Well illustrated.

23 **Cameron, M. and Hofvander, Y.**, *Manual on Feeding Infants and Young Children.* Protein Advisory Group of the UN, New York, PAG Document 1, 14/26, 1971, 239 pp. Intended for use in developing countries, with special reference to nutritious weaning foods, this manual contains 107 low-cost but nourishing recipes from countries around the world, which can be prepared locally. Information is given on the growth, development, and nutritional needs of children,

and on the values of different foods. Intended for all those concerned with the care of infants and young children, the manual aims to encourage the printing of local editions. A bibliography is included.

24 **Camrass, Rex,** *Western Samoa: Delivery of Dental Services in an Emergent Nation.* British Dental Journal, (London), Vol. 135 No. 7, October 1973, pp. 337–340. This article reports on the growth of a programme to provide dental services, involving mobile clinics, for the rural population in Western Samoa, with the cooperation of the local village committees. It includes suggestions for local inservice training and use of ancillary personnel both in preventive programmes and to provide treatment as part of a dental team.

25 **Canada, Department of National Health and Welfare,** *A Manual for Community Aides.* Department of National Health and Welfare, Ottawa, 1970, 15 pp. This manual, which lists common illnesses and the treatment of each, is intended for use by community aides in their day to day work. It also includes a section on the use of the radio for communication between community aides and doctors and nurses.

26 **Canada, Department of National Health and Welfare,** *A Sanitation Manual for*

Community Health Workers. Department of National Health and Welfare, Ottawa, (no date), 101 pp. Subjects covered in this manual, which is for use in Indian and Eskimo reserves, include basic principles of sanitation in relation to germs, disease, and water; the danger of disease spreading by several domestic insects and animals; and human waste disposal. The appendix gives a list of teaching materials on sanitation that are available from the Department, and a suggested programme for the community health worker. Useful.

27 **Canada, Department of National Health and Welfare,** *Family Health Manual.* Department of National Health and Welfare, Ottawa, (no date), 74 pp. This manual, which is addressed to Indians and Eskimos, covers the basic principles of hygiene and personal wellbeing, and relates them to stages in life such as adolescence and pregnancy. Separate chapters deal with family health, maternal and child health, dental hygiene, and the treatment of venereal diseases, rabies, etc.

28 **Canada, Department of National Health and Welfare,** *Mother and Baby.* Department of National Health and Welfare, Ottawa, 1972, 72 pp. In simple language, this booklet describes how a mother should look after herself and her baby, including feeding during the first twelve months of life. It contains forms

and charts to be filled by the mother and the doctor, and states when visits to the doctor should be made. The booklet is illustrated and should be useful for teaching.

29 **Church, Michael A.,** *Fluids for the Sick Child: A Method for Teaching Mothers.* Tropical Doctor, (London), Vol. 2, 1972, pp. 119–121. This article describes a regime used in Uganda whereby mothers learn, through active participation, how to rehydrate their sick children and prevent subsequent loss of fluids. A very useful article on an important subject in community health. •

30 **Colombia, Ministerio de Salud Publica,** *Manual Para el Adiestramiento de Promotoras Rurales de Salud (Manual for Teachers of Rural Health Care Workers).* Ministerio de Salud Publica, Division de Atencion Medica, Colombia, 1969, 237 pp. In Spanish. This manual covers many aspects of health care methods for rural health promoters, such as prevention of disease, the use of first-aid, maternal and child health, and health education. It describes the organisation and programme of an eight-week course for village health workers.

31 **Conference of Missionary Societies in Great Britain and Ireland,** *A Model Health Centre.* The Medical Committee of the Conference of Missionary Societies in Great Britain and Ireland, London, 1975, 170 pp.

The report shows how, with careful planning, a clinic can be developed into a health centre to provide health care for a population of up to 20,000 people. It describes the essentials of a health centre: under-fives clinic, pharmacy, laboratory, stores, equipment lists, communications, training, teaching aids, home visiting, costs, materials, buildings, treatment, etc. Very useful for anyone planning or involved in the delivery of health services to rural areas. Well illustrated with diagrams and drawings.

32 **Courtejoie, J. and Rotstart de Hertaing, I.,** *Manuel de Pharmacologie pour les Regions Tropicales a l'usage des Infirmiers et Infirmieres (Tropical Pharmacology Manual for Nurses).* Editions Saint Paul, Limete-Kinshasha, Zaire, 1971, 340 pp. In French. This manual of pharmacology for tropical regions is written for hospital attendants and for doctors teaching auxiliaries. It is a valuable and practical source book.

33 **Cox, Helen,** *Midwifery Manual: A Guide for Auxiliary Midwives.* McGraw-Hill International Health Series, Singapore, 1971, 240 pp. This very useful manual is intended for auxiliary midwives who are already skilled in normal midwifery. Its aim is to expand their potential in relation to the provision of good antenatal care and to guide them in the emergency action they may have

to undertake when medical assistance may not be immediately available. The book contains chapters on health teaching, family care, communicable diseases, family planning, elementary nursing, first aid, and health centre organization. This excellent book could be invaluable in helping auxiliary midwives to expand and extend their role.

34 Dean, Pauline, *Paediatric Out-Patients' Manual—Africa.* St. Luke's Hospital, Anua-Uyo, Nigeria. Also available from The Medical Missionaries of Mary, International Missionary Training Hospital, Drogheda, Eire, 1973, 50 pp. This extremely practical booklet is clearly and simply set out with useful index and tables including drug dosages for children. It is invaluable for training and as a reference book for auxiliaries in their daily work. The author is writing for student nurses but her philosophy is equally applicable to other similar health care personnel, and the value of health education and nutrition is stressed. Although written for Africa, this model ought to be adapted for other parts of the world.

35 Ebrahim, G. J., *Newborn in Tropical Africa.* East African Literature Bureau, Nairobi/Dar es Salaam, 1969, 111 pp. Also available from TALC (see entry 114). This review is excellent for medical students and paediatricians who deal with neonatal problems in the tropics.

It contains practical instructions on prenatal care, pregnancy disorders, midwifery, feeding, congenital defects, and the care of the newborn. It should be useful for teachers of medical auxiliaries at a fairly advanced level. Well illustrated, with an index and many references.

36 Ebrahim, G. J., *Child Care in the Tropics.* East African Literature Bureau, Nairobi/Dar es Salaam, 1971, 112 pp. Also available from TALC. As parents and teachers are responsible for the health, care, and nutrition of children in primary and secondary schools, this book is of value to them. It is also useful for medical auxiliaries working in community health and educational centres. It covers the newborn, infant nutrition, the development of the child, training, and diseases of children.

37 Ebrahim, G. J., *Practical Mother and Child Health in Developing Countries.* East African Literature Bureau, Nairobi/Dar es Salaam, 1973, 109 pp. Also available from TALC. This simply presented book discusses methods and services necessary for the health of mother and child. It provides useful background information for all medical workers, and practical hints for medical auxiliaries and midwives in particular. A very useful book in all areas of maternal and child health work.

8

38 **Essex, B. J.,** *Diagnostic Pathways in Clinical Medicine—An Epidemiological Approach to Clinical Problems.* Churchill Livingstone, Edinburgh/London/New York, 1977, 173 pp. The aim of this book is to provide paramedical workers and young doctors with skills needed to make an accurate diagnosis in the outpatient clinic, in less than 3 minutes per patient. It is based upon scientific methods which have been tested for accuracy, usefulness, and economy. The book covers modern ideas about the causes of disease, disease patterns and outpatient problems, the skills of outpatient diagnosis, description of some important physical signs, flow charts and disease tables, evaluation studies, and the problems of outpatient management. Although developed specifically for East African regions, the book could be useful for other areas.

39 **Fensom, M.,** *Midwifery* One of a series: Oxford Handbooks for Medical Auxiliaries. Oxford University Press, London, 1971, 94 pp. This elementary manual on midwifery, written in simple language, covers concepts easily grasped by novices. It is written for midwives in developing countries and for teachers of traditional birth attendants, and is suitable for translation into the vernacular. Covers the practical essentials of maternity care. Illustrated.

40 **Fountain, Daniel E.,** *The Art of Diagnosis for Medical Assistants.* Lange Medical Publications, Los Altos, California, 1974, 206 pp. Written for students in the final year of a 3-year medical auxiliary training programme in Zaire, this illustrated booklet should also be useful for teachers as a source book. It covers in detail such topics as: how to make a diagnosis; symptom diagnosis; community diagnosis.

41 **Gally, Esther,** *Manual practico para parteras (Practical Manual for Midwives).* Editorial Pax-Mexico, Mexico City, 1977, 559 pp. In Spanish. This manual, which is written for health workers with or without formal technical training, covers antenatal care, management of labour, and postnatal care. It emphasizes the provision of family planning and midwifery services within the rural community. Guidelines for history taking, examination diagnosis, medical referral and treatment, and child care are included. Extensively illustrated with diagrams and photographs.

42 **Gally, Esther,** *Planificacion Familiar Es Bienestar (Family Planning is Well-Being).* Editorial Pax-Mexico, Mexico City, (no date). In Spanish. This 14-sheet full colour flipchart with special text for instructor on back of every page is very useful for social and health workers in family planning clinics. Developed with the Mexican Ministry of Health, the

flipchart is being used throughout Latin America for motivating and informing patients. A booklet by the same name is available for distribution to reinforce the family planning message.

43   Goarnisson, J. and Blanc, C., *Guide Médical Africain, Médicine Tropicale.* Editions Saint Paul, Issy-les-Moulieaux, France, 1972, 743 pp. In French. This book is suitable for use as a manual for medical assistants and families who might be responsible for the care of the community's health. It deals with illnesses common to tropical countries, particularly in Africa, and indicates causes, symptoms and treatment for each disease. It also covers the examination of the patient, medical and surgical techniques, emergency cases, skin diseases, child pathology, etc. Several illustrations and a subject index are included.

44   Gonzales, William V., *Manual de Procedimientos para el Asistente de Salud Rural (Manual of Procedures for the Rural Health Assistant).* Ministry of Health, San Jose, Costa Rica, 1972, 118 pp. Also available in English and French from WHO (see entry 138). Addressed to villagers selected to be health workers in their community after limited training, this is a reference text. It covers nursing procedures, home visits, vaccination, hygiene, first aid, maternal and child health, environmental

sanitation, and identification of the most common diseases. The appendix covers the use and administration of drugs.

45   Gray, Herman H., *Treatment Handbook for Health Centres in West Africa.* Christian Council of Nigeria, Ikot Ibritam, Nigeria, 1973, 58 pp. Intended for dispensary attendants and midwives in West Africa, this manual gives descriptions of various diseases. It covers maintenance of the dispensary and maternity home, team work, care of the sick, health education, children's drug dosages, etc. It also covers preventive health: vaccines, family planning, and special instructions for midwives.

46   Halestrap, David J., *Simple Dental Care for Rural Hospitals.* Medical Missionary Association, London, 1971, 26 pp. Also available from TALC (see entry 114). This booklet is intended as a guide for dental auxiliary workers in developing countries. It is illustrated with line drawings and photographs which have been pre-tested to make them appropriate for the auxiliary, and the language is simplified for workers who use English as a second language.

47   Hamza, M. H. and Segall, Malcolm N., *Care of the Newborn Baby in Tanzania.* Tanzania Publishing House, Dar es Salaam, 1973, 43 pp. Also available from TALC. This manual was written for

Tanzanian medical assistants, but nurses, rural medical aides, medical students and doctors should find it useful. It gives an account of the most important aspects of care of newborn babies. It also describes common abnormalities and their treatment, and the care of low birth-weight babies. Very useful. Excellent line drawings.

48   Harnar, R., Cummins, A., Arole, R. S., and Arole, M., *Teaching Village Health Workers—a Guide to the Process.* Voluntary Health Association of India, New Delhi, 1978, 120 pp. This comprehensive pack is a guide to the teaching of village health workers (VHWs) which includes two books and many simple audio-visual aids. One guide book covers the concepts and planning of teaching VHWs, and the other contains curriculum charts and lesson plans. Practical aspects and problems encountered in teaching VHWs are emphasized throughout, and the simple aids can be adapted for local use and production. It is an excellent model for adaptation elsewhere.

49   Hay, R. W. and Whitehead, R. G., *The Therapy of the Severely Malnourished Child.* National Food and Nutrition Council of Uganda in Collaboration with the M.R.C. Child Nutrition Unit, Kampala, 1973, 47 pp. Primarily intended for use in Uganda, this booklet is addressed to doctors and medical assistants involved in treating severely malnourished children. It gives details of diets, costs of food, and management of various problems in clear and simple tables, and has many illustrations.

50   Hoff, P. H. Wilbur, *The Importance of Training for Effective Performance.* Public Health Reports, (Washington), Vol. 85, No. 9, 1970, pp. 760–766. Adequate training probably contributes more than any other factor to the successful performance of auxiliary health workers. The article outlines components of the training of health aides including identifying health problems, providing personal health care, and performing general administrative duties and basic educational functions. The author emphasizes the need to train supervisors and trainers of health aides. A short outline of a training programme is included with references, and a selected annotated bibliography on health aides is given.

51   Hopwood, B. E. C. and Lovel, H. J., *The Wallo Exercise: Planning for Rural Health Services in Africa—Organisers' Manual and Participants' Manual.* Commonwealth Secretariat, London, 1975, 30 pp. These two documents outline an exercise in practical health planning for a hypothetical typical African country, designed for medical staff who may be involved in health services administration. Participants are expected to

11

organize themselves to produce proposals for the arrangement and distribution of health facilities in the imaginary Wallo area, for which geographical, economic and other data are given. Suitable only for district medical officers, project officers, and coordinators.

52   **India, Ministry of Health and Family Welfare,** *Manual for Community Health Workers.* Ministry of Health and Family Welfare, New Delhi, 1977, 154 pp. The manual has been prepared for Community Health Workers, (CHWs), now being trained in the primary health centres all over India. It contains information on the fundamentals of health, treatment of common ailments, maternal and child welfare, first aid, communicable diseases, nutrition, and mental health. Special care has been taken to see that the CHWs obtain fundamental knowledge about the traditional systems of medicine, yoga, ayurveda, unani and siddha, and homeopathy, which they should utilise for the improvement of the health of the people. Useful appendices are included.

53   **India, Rural Health Research Centre,** *Standing Orders for the Care of Sick Children.* Rural Health Research Centre (R.H.R.C.), Narangwal, India, 1972, 30 pp. This document gives indications for referrals to doctors by community health workers. It then lists very comprehensively various diseases and abnormalities, giving their symptoms, and explains how to examine patients and take down case histories. Treatment is then described, and so is follow-up routine, with instructions when to refer to a doctor. Though a good basic reminder guide, it is not teaching material as such, but could very usefully supplement such material.

54   **Indian Academy of Paediatricians,** *Health Care of Children Under Five: Report of a Workshop of the Indian Academy of Paediatricians, Institute of Child Health, Hyderabad, and the Voluntary Health Association of India.* McGraw Hill, Bombay, 1973, 98 pp. Also available from TALC (see entry 114). This detailed discussion of organization of under-five clinics includes ground plans, use of the 'Road to Health' chart, immunization schedules, and 'Standing Orders for Treatment'. It emphasizes health education, and is suitable for all those involved with under-five clinics.

55   **Indonesia, Lembaga Kesehatan Nasional,** *The Child in the Health Centre.* Lembaga Kesehatan Nasional, Jalan Indrapura, Indonesia, 1974, 554 pp. This detailed, illustrated manual of health centre paediatrics is an experimental edition written in basic English as part of a child care package. It aims to serve both as a text for training schools and as a manual for use in the clinic afterwards.

It should be useful for many countries in addition to Indonesia.

56   **Indonesia,** *Health Care Reference Manual.* Directorate General of Community Health, Jakarta, 1976. This manual, in four volumes, aims to serve as both an information reference source and daily practical guide for health centre staff in Indonesia. Its 14 sections cover topics ranging from administration and management, health education, and nutrition, to communicable disease control and technical laboratory procedures. Numerous charts, diagrams, and photographs complement the manual's detailed information, which is arranged for quick access by health workers.

57   **International Development Research Centre,** *Health Care in the People's Republic of China.* Edited by Shahid Akhtar, IDRC, Ottawa, 1974, 182 pp. Of interest to planners and those concerned with training health workers, this book includes materials on planning, financing and organization of health care systems. It discusses the impact of health care services on social and economic indices, the relationships between health care systems and other community organization and staffing.

58   **Jancloes, M.,** *Manuel Pratique pour Infirmiers de Dispensaires Ruraux (Practical Manual for Rural Dispensary Workers).* Centre Medical de Kisantu, Inkisi, Zaire, 1974, 68 pp. In French. This manual is intended for the use of rural dispensary nurses who are receiving further training. It is practical and based on the experience these health workers already possess. It revises existing knowledge, augments this, and shows ways to promote health education and preventive care in rural areas. Useful for teachers of auxiliaries.

59   **Jelliffe, D. B.,** *Child Nutrition in Developing Countries.* U.S. Department of Health, Education and Welfare, Washington, 1968, 169 pp. This book is written simply for those who have had no previous training in the health field. It outlines general principles of child nutrition and the causes, symptoms, and treatment of malnutrition. Sources of necessary nutrients in tropical foods, weight for age, and sample weaning recipes from various parts of the world are also included. Excellent source-book for teachers.

60   **Jelliffe, D. B.,** *Child Health in the Tropics.* Edward Arnold, London, 1974, 170 pp. This practical and simple book is intended for use by medical and paramedical personnel, and particularly by their teachers. It covers the clinical, preventive, and social aspects of child health in the tropics, as well as nutritional deficiencies, diarrhoeal diseases, infections, and health education. It also

contains a useful list of paediatric drug dosages, a suggested schedule of immunization, a valuable bibliography, and an index. Illustrated with line drawings.

61 **John E. Fogarty International Center for Advanced Study in the Health Sciences,** Barefoot Doctor's Manual. U.S. Department of Health, Education, and Welfare, Public Health Service, Washington, 1974, 960 pp. This manual is divided into seven chapters which cover hygiene, diagnostic and therapeutic techniques, birth control, common disorders, and Chinese medicinal plants. It integrates Western medicine and traditional Chinese medicine, with emphasis on the Chinese. About 522 illustrated herbs are listed and many tested prescriptions based on their effectiveness are given. The manual focuses on the improvement of medical and health care facilities in the rural villages, aiming through local adaptation to meet the working needs of barefoot doctors serving the rural population.

62 **Jopling, W. H.,** Handbook of Leprosy. Heinemann Medical Books Ltd., London, 1971, 99 pp. This handbook provides basic information for use by health workers in areas where leprosy is endemic. It describes in simple and concise terms the diagnosis, classification, treatment, and management of leprosy. It also lists the types of

drugs which may be given to patients. A glossary of terms and an index are included.

63 **Keister, M. E.,** Child Care, A Handbook for Village Workers and Leaders. Food and Agriculture Organization, Rome, 1971, 58 pp. Intended for anyone interested in child care, this handbook covers hygiene, nutrition, immunization and parental involvement. It gives practical ideas on learning activities and teaching aids.

64 **Khita, M. B. et al.,** La Jeunesse et Problèmes des Naissances Desirables (Youth and the Problem of Planned Births). Bureau d'Etudes et de Recherches pour la Promotion de la Santé, Kangu, Zaire, 1974, 51 pp. In French. This book contains sex education and birth control information, written simply but comprehensively. It emphasizes clearly the happiness of the planned family. Although in French, it could be adapted for use in other countries. Illustrated with photographs and diagrams.

65 **King, Maurice,** (editor), Medical Care in Developing Countries. Oxford University Press, Nairobi/London, 1966. Spanish edition available from Editorial Pax-Mexico, Mexico City. Based on a UNICEF-assisted conference, this work contains practical advice on many aspects of medical care in developing countries, such as planning and organization of the health

services, the running of a health centre, the role of the auxiliary, teaching aids, etc. It deals with diagnosis briefly, and with treatment in detail. Several references, a bibliography, and details of drug dosages are included. Very useful for all categories of health personnel.

66   **King, Maurice and King, F.,** *Nutrition in Developing Countries.* Oxford University Press, Nairobi/London, 1972, 325 pp. Also available from TALC (see entry 114). This book is meant particularly for the maize, cassava and millet growing areas of Africa, but much of it would be useful in other areas. It is simply written for the training of medical assistants, medical students, nurses and midwives, community development workers and cadres of rural workers in health and development. It covers the nutritional diagnosis of a community, how to initiate a community health programme, and how to supervise the nutrition of children using the age-for-weight charts. It aims also to help mothers understand the fundamentals of child nutrition, supplementary feeding, the value of certain foods, etc. Well illustrated.

67   **King, Maurice,** *A Medical Laboratory for Developing Countries.* Oxford Medical Publications, Oxford, 1973, 380 pp. Spanish edition available from Editorial Pax-Mexico, Mexico City.

Written in simple English, this book aims to bring basic pathological services to everyone in developing countries. Each piece of equipment needed in a medical laboratory is fully described and illustrated with detailed drawings. Every step in the examination of specimens is simply explained, and methods of obtaining specimens are described. Where necessary, anatomy, physiology, and a brief account of treatment are included. The last chapter gives a detailed equipment list, and there are numerous drawings and colour plates. Invaluable as a model for similar books covering other health fields.

68   **Koppert, Joan,** *The Nutrition Rehabilitation Village.* The National Food and Nutrition Commission, Lusaka, 1972, 25 pp. Also available from TALC. This practical and down-to-earth book on the planning and organization of nutrition rehabilitation programmes covers topics such as financing, staff selection, diets, record-keeping and evaluation. It emphasizes the involvement of mothers in the programme so that they can learn while tending to their children and thus transfer good nutrition and health ideas to the community. The book is useful for workers involved in maternal child health, health education, and community development programmes, and subjects such as the preparation of food, home gardening, enlisting parental cooperation, etc. are also

included. Well illustrated with diagrams and photographs. References included.

69 Koppert, Joan, *A Guide to Nutrition Rehabilitation.* 'Contact' 23, (Geneva), 1974, 16 pp. This very useful guide for setting up a nutrition rehabilitation centre includes staffing, daily activities, and dietary instructions. It emphasizes that health and growth are not related to medicine but to eating an adequate quantity of food. The author considers that a medical assistant could well be in overall charge of such a centre.

70 La Liberté, Dolores (editor), *Child Health Care in Rural Areas —A Manual for Auxiliary Nurse Midwives.* Asia Publishing House, Bombay, 1974, 363 pp. Also available from TALC (see entry 114). In this manual, for use during training and for reference at primary health centres in India, diagnosis is dealt with at a simple level and treatment is dealt with extensively. It includes tables of drugs and dosages, and has good clear illustrations. The manual could easily be adapted for other countries and for use by medical auxiliaries.

71 Latham, M., *Human Nutrition in Tropical Africa.* FAO, Rome, 1965, 240 pp. Also available in French. This book is designed to assist health workers in East Africa to diagnose and solve the nutritional problems of their communities. Topics covered include basic nutrition, community health aspects of nutrition, malnutrition, diet, home preservation of food, etc. The appendices include recommended intakes of nutrients, food composition tables, and a list of references. A good source book for teachers, it is well illustrated and also applicable for regions outside Africa.

72 Laugesen, Helen, *Better Child Care.* Voluntary Health Association of India, New Delhi, 1977, 52 pp. This booklet covers the basic problems and illnesses of childhood, and gives practical solutions for prevention and treatment at village level. It is a series of pre-tested photographs with a simply written text for use as a teaching and memory aid by field workers. Photographs for diagnosis of undernutrition, anaemia, and Vitamin A deficiency are included, and information on antenatal care, childbirth, nutritional needs of the child, management of common childhood illnesses, etc. is given. The booklet's small size makes it especially suitable for field use, and it could be used for producing other teaching materials for training auxiliaries and village health workers and for community education.

73 Lucas, A. O. and Gilles, H. M., *A Short Textbook of Preventive Medicine for the Tropics.* English Universities Press, Kent, 1973, 326 pp. This introduction to the concepts of

16

preventive medicine is written for medical students in developing countries. It covers a wide area clearly and concisely, and much of the material is sufficiently basic to be of use for auxiliary teaching.

74   **Malawi, Department of Extension and Training,** *A Guide to Health and Good Food for the Family.* Department of Extension and Training, Ministry of Agriculture and Natural Resources, Lilongwe, Malawi, 1975, 57 pp. Also available in Chichewa. Simply written, with good illustrations, this book is particularly for rural families, schools, and women's groups. It could be useful for trainers and auxiliaries working in the field with the community. Covers nutrition, hygiene, environmental sanitation, communicable diseases. There is also a section on useful recipes for weaning foods, and for meals for children and invalids.

75   **Malawi, Ministry of Health,** *Handbook for Medical Assistants for Use in Rural Health Units.* Compiled by Robertson, Katherine M., Ministry of Health, Malawi, 1969, 130 pp. This handbook is designed to serve as a guide for Medical Assistants working in Rural Health Units throughout Malawi. It deals with diseases and ailments commonly seen, and the diagnosis and treatments given can easily be undertaken at such units. The handbook is divided into sections such as disorders of the alimentary

system, diseases of the respiratory system, childbirth and disorders in women, infectious diseases, disorders affecting the nervous system, nutritional disorders, eye diseases, diseases of the skin, and surgical conditions. Useful appendices are included.

76   **Malaysia, Ministry of Health,** *Training Programmes for Para-Medical and Auxiliary Staff.* Division of Training and Manpower, Ministry of Health, Kuala Lumpur, 1975, 26 pp. This booklet gives details of training centres, entry requirements, and outlines of courses provided in Malaysia for various categories of paramedical and auxiliary staff such as the public health inspector, state registered nurse, radiographer, dental nurse, public health visitor, nurse midwife, junior laboratory assistant, assistant nurse, etc.

77   **Malaysia, Ministry of Health,** *The Training of Student Midwives for Part II of the Register (Sukatan Pelajaran Untuk Lathihan Bidan Bahagian II).* Ministry of Health, Kuala Lumpur, May 1976, 9 pp. This syllabus for the training of student midwives covers nursing, anatomy and physiology, midwifery and the problems of abnormal pregnancies. The training lasts 24 months, 18 months of which are spent in a hospital, and the remaining 6 months in domestic accommodation. The course covers health education,

maternal child health, rural health, environmental sanitation, and communicable diseases.

78   **Mehra, June D.**, *Localised Production of Communication Materials —The Baroda Project.* UNICEF, New Delhi, 1977, 60 pp. This report discusses the evolution of a communication strategy to produce communication materials by involving (and thereby training) government personnel at the state, district, and block levels, together with village people, to produce communication materials on nutrition, health, and child care. The materials are specifically related to the needs and conditions of the villagers of Chota Udaipur tribal block, India, with particular reference to their food habits and taboos. The paper includes various pre-testing and evaluation procedures used, and the results obtained. Illustrated. Very useful.

79   **Nepal, Family Planning and Maternal Child Health Project,** *A Working Manual for Clinical FP/MCH: Activities for Use by Junior Paramedical Workers.* Family Planning and Maternal Child Health Project of the Nepal Government, Kathmandu, February 1976, 12 pp. This useful step-by-step symptom treatment manual covers the most common maternal and child health problems of rural communities. It emphasizes the use of low-cost

equipment, and is simply written. Very useful.

80   **Nepal, Health Ministry,** *Health Post Technical Staff—Operations Manual.* Department of Health Services, Kathmandu, 1975, 200 pp. Written in simple English, this illustrated manual could be useful for all categories of health workers. It is a good reference guide for trainers of auxiliaries and for health post workers. Detailed coverage is given to infectious diseases and their control, family planning, maternal and child health, and nutrition, but environmental sanitation is only covered briefly. A separate section on the auxiliary nurse midwife is included, giving details on home visiting, domiciliary midwifery, and midwifery emergencies.

81   **Nestlé Company Limited,** *Standard Treatments for Common Illnesses of Children in Papua New Guinea.* The Nestlé Company (Australia) Ltd, Sydney, 1974, 48 pp. This pocket-sized manual is a good reference guide for nurses, extension officers or rural doctors, for the effective standard treatment of common illnesses in children—such as anaemia, diarrhoea, malnutrition, low birth weight, etc. It contains simple treatments and adequate information on symptoms and diagnosis. Very useful.

82   **Oxfam,** *Memorandum on Tuberculosis Control in*

Developing Countries. Oxfam, Oxford, 1971, 20 pp. Also available from TALC (see entry 114). This is a clear and concise survey of the extent of the tuberculosis problem and principles of treatment. It emphasizes the importance of planning in tuberculosis control campaigns.

83 **Papua New Guinea, Department of Public Health,** *Our Patients: A Study for Health Workers.* Nursing Education Division of Department of Public Health, Konedobu, (no date). This illustrated text deals with human biology and simple disease conditions met with in elementary nursing and aid-post management. It is written specifically for use in Papua New Guinea.

84 **Papua New Guinea, Department of Public Health,** *Midwifery Manual for Community Nurses.* Maternal and Child Health Section, Department of Public Health, Port Moresby, 1970, 175 pp. Reproduced by WHO 1974 (see entry 136). This manual is intended for nurses working in well equipped specialised units of a centrally organised health service, recommendations for treatment in a village situation being limited to first aid measures and referral to hospitals. The text includes basic anatomy, female reproductive system, obstetric operations, and a brief outline of family planning methods. It also covers care of

the newborn, lists of obstetric drugs and definitions, and various procedures in the labour ward.

85 **Papua New Guinea, Department of Public Health,** *Drug Reference for Nurses.* Division of Medical Training, Department of Public Health, Konedobu, 1974, 259 pp. Written for nurses, this extremely clear reference book contains tables of abbreviations used for drug dosages, tables for calculating dosages, and drawings of equipment for drug administration. It lists drugs according to the route by which they are given, and gives some dosage schedules.

86 **Papua New Guinea, Paramedical College.** Further details of the following documents can be obtained from the Paramedical College, Madang.
The Diseases and Health Services of Papua New Guinea. Edited by Clive Bell, Port Moresby, 1973.
Medical and Paramedical Training in Papua New Guinea. Division of Medical Training, Department of Public Health.
Environmental Health and Sanitation. Beri, K. K. et al., 1972.
Child Health-Nutrition and Growth. Student Workbook, Teacher's Guide.
Obstetrics for Nursing Aides Nursing Aide Manual Obstetrical and Gynaecological Problems in the Highlands of New Guinea

Look After Your Hands and Feet (Leprosy) Aid Post Orderly Workshop 28 May 1973-1 June 1973.

87   **Pasnik, Judith L.,** *Reference and Training Manual for Physical Therapy Technicians in Leprosy.* American Leprosy Missions Inc., New York, (no date), 134 pp. Addressed to physical therapy technicians and therefore not directly for auxiliaries, this is nevertheless a very useful source book for instructors and potential authors of textbooks for auxiliaries. Well illustrated.

88   **Peru, Ministerio de Salud Publica,** *Manual of Standards and Procedures for Nursing Auxiliaries in Health Posts in the Puno Health Area.* Ministerio de Salud Publica, Lima, 1967, in Spanish. Reproduced in English and French by WHO, 1973, 164 pp. (see entry 135). Addressed to auxiliaries working in rural health posts in Puno, Peru, this manual is written in simple language and explains the functions and duties of the village health worker. Most common diseases and the application of first aid are described. It emphasizes the importance of administrative practices such as registration of births, deaths, etc., and provides a list of minimum supplies required for a health post, including samples of reporting forms for the centre. Well

illustrated. References included. Useful and comprehensive.

89   **Philippines, Family Planning Organisation,** Training Handbooks: *Why the Philippines needs Family Planning, Medical Handbook, IUD Handbook, Casebook on Oral Contraceptives, How to Begin a Family Planning Programme.* Family Planning Organisation of the Philippines, Manila, approx. 80 pp. each. Although possibly too technical in places for auxiliaries, these illustrated books could provide useful background material for trainers that could be adapted to local situations.

90   **Philpott, R. H. and Sapire, K. E.,** *Obstetrics, Family Planning and Paediatrics: a Manual of Practical Management for Doctors and Nurses.* Family Planning Association of Rhodesia, Salisbury, (no date), 106 pp. The authors of this manual for doctors and nurses, aware of the problems of high birthrate and high maternal and infant mortality in developing countries, maintain that obstetric, family planning, and paediatric services should be integrated. They have therefore incorporated these subjects into 3 detailed sections. There are lists of useful drugs and dosages, and the treatment and measures taken to prevent kwashiorkor and other debilitating diseases prevalent in Third World countries are covered. Also

included are a weight chart and an immunization plan.

91 Planned Parenthood World Population, *Family Planning, A Teaching Guide for Nurses.* Planned Parenthood World Population, New York, 1969, 86 pp. Also available in French, 1971, 82 pp. This guide is intended for nursing-school teachers and for nurses responsible for education in their communities. Topics covered include the history of family planning, population problems, birth control, poverty, anatomy and physiology of reproduction, methods of birth control, etc. It also includes a bibliography. A useful source book for teachers.

92 Reid, S. E. and Johnson, D. G., *Obstetrics for Health Extension Officers.* University of Papua New Guinea, Port Moresby, 1972, 154 pp. This manual provides health extension officers in Papua New Guinea with information on the provision of obstetric care. It covers anatomy, antenatal care, normal and abnormal childbirth, and complications of pregnancy and labour. All symptoms are simply explained with clear line drawings, and a comprehensive glossary and index are included.

93 Rogoff, M., *Laboratory Assistant's Manual.* McGraw-Hill International Publications Co. Ltd., London, 1974, 208 pp. The book is intended specifically for the laboratory assistant in inaccessible areas of developing countries, who has to produce accurate results under very difficult conditions. The book contains the accumulated experience of many years in the field of laboratory medicine in Central and East Africa, and includes procedures suitable for rural laboratories. It is clearly written, well illustrated and excellent value.

94 Rohde, Jon Eliot and Northrup, Robert S., *Mother as the Basic Health Worker— Training her and her Trainers.* Presented at Bellagio Consultation: New Type of Basic Health Services World Wide and the Implication for the Education of other Health Care Professionals, 2–7 May, 1977, 40 pp. This paper describes health problems in Indonesia and a new approach involving 7,000 family planning field workers and millions of mothers in a highly organized outreach effort to bring maternal and child health care into every child's home. Tasks and actions to be carried out by mothers are clearly defined, and special teaching materials have been designed. Intensive promotion is carried out, and the linkage with a new curriculum for medical students is a valuable example for other countries with similar problems.

95 Rosinski, E. F. and Spencer, F. J., *El Auxiliar Medico (The Medical Auxiliary).* Editorial Pax-Mexico, Mexico City, 1974. In Spanish. This is an outline of training programmes concerned with both prevention and treatment of illness, and all other aspects of health promotion.

96 **Rotsart de Hertaing, I.** et al., *Education Nutritionnelle (Nutrition Education).* Bureau d'Etudes et de Recherches pour la Promotion de la Santé, Kangu, Zaire, (no date), 22 pp. In French. The value of 'Road to Health' weight charts is emphasized in this booklet, which provides a sensible guide to nutrition education. The recommendations are practical and the authors stress the need to begin educating girls very early in the principles of nutrition. A very useful book for everyone involved in maternal and child health care.

97 **Rotsart de Hertaing, I.** et al., *La Jeunesse et les Maladies Vénériennes (Adolescence and Venereal Diseases).* Bureau d'Etudes et de Recherches pour la Promotion de la Santé, Kangu, Zaire, 1974, 23 pp. In French. This booklet is moderately technical but within the understanding of anyone with secondary school education. A useful book for medical auxiliaries and their teachers. Good illustrations.

98 **Rotsart de Hertaing, I.** et al., *La Médicine à L'Ecole (School Health).* Bureau d'Etudes et de Recherches pour la Promotion de la Santé, Kangu, Zaire, 1974, 23 pp. In French. This booklet aims at promoting better contacts between schools, hospitals and dispensaries through regular medical examination of school children combined with health education teaching in the schools, and active involvement of the pupils in all health-related activities. Well illustrated and full of interesting ideas.

99 **Rotsart de Hertaing, I.** et al., *La Santé de vos Enfants (Your Children's Health).* Bureau d'Etudes et de Recherches pour la Promotion de la Santé, Kangu, Zaire, 1974, 47 pp. In French. This booklet is intended for parents who want to know more about the care of their young children. It gives simple explanations of the value of preventive measures and the way to deal with childhood illnesses. Useful for auxiliaries as a basis for family health education.

100 **Rotsart de Hertaing, I.** et al., *Education de la Santé dans l'Enseignement Primaire et Secondaire (Health Education in Primary and Secondary Schools).* Bureau d'Etudes et de Recherches pour la Promotion de la Santé, Kangu, (no date), 31 pp. In French. The authors suggest methods of promoting better health among school children by integrating health education into the school curriculum in both primary and secondary schools. The booklet has novel suggestions e.g. the arithmetic class can calculate the answers to nutritional and other health-related problems. Imaginative and very useful for teachers.

101 Rotsart de Hertaing, I. and Courtejoie, J., *L'Education Sanitaire (Health Education).* Bureau d'Etudes et de Recherches pour la Promotion de la Santé, Kangu, Zaire, 1974, 35 pp. In French. The authors emphasize that curative and preventive medicine and health education are inseparable parts of the responsibility of all doctors and nurses working in the community. The booklet contains very useful guidelines for devising health education programmes suitable for different age groups. Suitable for auxiliaries and for teachers of auxiliaries. Well illustrated.

102 Ross Institute of Tropical Hygiene. The Institute publishes a very useful series of Bulletins, some of which are reviewed separately in this bibliography. Many are suitable for teachers of auxiliaries. Titles in the series include:
Malaria and its Control. Bruce-Chwatt, L. J.
Protein Calorie Malnutrition in Children. Burgess, J. J. L.
Rural Sanitation in the Tropics. Davidson, G.
Anaemia in the Tropics. Wadworth, G. R.
Schistosomiasis. Southgate, B. A.
A complete list may be obtained from the Ross Institute, London.

103 Royal Tropical Institute. In conjunction with WHO, the Institute publishes a series of visual aids and texts which are suitable for medical auxiliaries. The series deals with the diagnosis and therapy of common diseases, and is meant to serve as an aid in the communication and teaching process between doctor and medical auxiliary. The titles in the series include:
Leprosy. Leiker, D. L., booklet with 48 slides.
Skin diseases. Klokke, A. H., booklet with 36 slides.
Eye diseases. Oosterhuis, J. A. and Franken, S., booklet with 36 slides.
Malnutrition. Oomen, H. A. P. C., booklet with 24 slides.
Ear, Nose and Throat diseases. Wind, J., illustrated booklet.
A complete list can be obtained from the Royal Tropical Institute, Amsterdam.

104 Rural Missionaries of the Philippines, *Guide for Community Health Programme.* Rural Missionaries of the Philippines Health Team, Manila, 1976, 101 pp. This guide has been prepared to assist those professional health workers who are willing to share their medical knowledge and skills with people. It is a collection of materials intended to stimulate sensitivity to the health needs of the community and to encourage creative responses in meeting those needs. The guide contains a description of a training programme and notes on a seminar. It includes some interesting papers on basic principles for a community-based health programme, expectations and relationships of village health workers, background data on health in the Philippines, and references.

105 **Rural Missionaries of the Philippines,** *Manual for Community Health Worker.* Rural Missionaries of the Philippines Health Team, Manila, 1976, 78 pp. This manual provides community health workers with handy reference information about the principles of good health and the nature and causes of disease. It contains information on nutrition, maternal and child health, first aid, transmission of disease, body systems, common childhood diseases, mental health, home nursing, environment and sanitation, immunization, medicines, and record forms used by community health workers. Illustrated with appropriate and simple drawings. Concise and useful.

106 **Schweser, H. O'Brien,** *A Manual for Community Health Education for the Caribbean.* The People-to-People Health Foundation Inc., Washington, 1976, 251 pp. The manual emphasizes that community participation is absolutely necessary for improving public health, and that health education is the means by which this cooperation can be obtained. It includes discussions of the role of doctors, nurses and auxiliaries in health education, and the role of workers in allied disciplines. It has an extensive bibliography.

107 **Shakir, A. and Morley, D.,** *Measuring Malnutrition.* Available from TALC (see entry 114). Reprinted from *The Lancet,* 20 April, 1974, 1 pp. This article describes the use of a three-coloured strip to measure mid-upper-arm circumference, which serves as a simple and reliable indicator of nutritional status in children up to 5 years. Very useful for quick surveys of *nutritional status of children in communities.*

108 **Standard, K. L. and Ennever, Olive,** *Manual for Community Health Workers.* Department of Social and Preventive Medicine, University of the West Indies, Kingston, (no date), 231 pp. Prepared by a team of doctors, nurses and social scientists for the training of community health workers in 3 months, this manual is very useful for any organization wanting to train auxiliaries. It is written in simple language with appropriate illustrations, and covers nutrition, basic nursing, personal hygiene, community health, environmental health, maternal and infant care, emotional problems of adults and children, etc.

109 **Stead, William W.,** *Understanding Tuberculosis Today: A Handbook for Patients.* Marquette University Press, Milwaukee, Wisconsin, 1971, 32 pp. This handbook, which gives simple up-to-date facts on the nature, diagnosis and treatment of tuberculosis (TB), discusses the four stages of

24

TB and how it can be detected. It contains hospital and out-patient treatment, a list of drugs most commonly used, preventive measures, and several case histories. Appended are notes, summaries, diagrams, clear and colourful cartoons, and a TB quiz.

110   **Stein, H. A. and Slatt, B. J.,** *The Ophthalmic Assistant.* C. V. Mosby Co. Ltd., St Louis, U.S.A., 1971, 470 pp. This basic reference source is written for the ophthalmic assistant who may not have had any formal training but learnt his skills 'on the job'. It includes sections on basic sciences, clinical practice including ocular emergencies, special procedures, community ocular problems, and an atlas of common eye disorders. It is clearly presented, written in good clear English, and could be used by teachers and auxiliaries fluent in English.

111   **St. John Ambulance Association,** *First Aid.* St. John Ambulance Association, London, 1972, 210 pp. This illustrated booklet is presented in a step-by-step format, with theoretical and practical instructions for each topic. It deals with the principles of first aid, emergency action, wounds and circulatory failure, injuries to bones, muscles, joints, burns, scalds, etc., and includes an index.

112   **Tanzania, Medical Assistants' Training Centre,** *Obstetrics and Gynaecology for*

Medical Assistants. Edited by Tengve, B., Medical Assistants' Training Centre, Bumbuli, Tanzania. Also from Vuga Press, Soni, Tanzania, 1973, 242 pp. This manual is intended for Tanzanian Medical Assistants' work in the field. It gives symptoms and treatment in simple words so that they can manage on their own in health centres. The value of health education and recording full medical histories is stressed. The syllabus is given, also emergencies and decisions for hospital referral. It suggests that Training Centre teachers adapt the manual to their local conditions where necessary.

113   **Tanzania, Ministry of Health,** *Mwanza Programme on Public Health. Second Half-yearly Report for 1973.* Ministry of Health, Dar es Salaam, 1974, 7 pp. The constantly evolving curriculum of medical auxiliaries related to the Mwanza public health programme, which started in 1969, is outlined. The programme is predominantly a public health teaching scheme in various schools for medical auxiliaries, which introduces public health administration concepts into continuing education programmes for rural health workers and supervisors.

114   **Teaching Aids at Low Cost (TALC).** TALC distributes inexpensive books and materials required by health workers. It produces a series of colour-slide sets for teaching, which covers

topics on nutrition, child health, infectious diseases, and family planning. Slide tape sets, slide tape tutors, and slide tape projectors are also available. A complete list of these teaching aids may be obtained from TALC, Institute of Child Health, London.

115   U.S.A., Department of Agriculture, *Homemaking Handbook for Village Workers in Many Countries.* Published in conjunction with U.S. Agency for International Development, Washington, 1971, 234 pp. Useful for any personnel working in community development, this handbook describes subjects such as food and nutrition, child care, health, agriculture, and home improvement and management. It illustrates some concepts by stories, and also discusses planning village programmes and teaching methods. A bibliography is appended.

116   U.S.A., Department of Health, Education and Welfare, *Health Auxiliary Training: Instructor's Guide.* Division of Indian Health, U.S. Department of Health, Education and Welfare, Washington, 1966, 273 pp. This manual gives a comprehensive outline for lectures and quizzes for training health auxiliaries. It was designed especially to channel personnel for comprehensive health programmes from among the population to be served, and in this case particularly among the American Indian and Alaska Natives.

117   van der Heyden, A., Courtejoie, J., Rotsart de Hertaing, I., *Les Vers Intestinaux (Intestinal Worms).* Bureau d'Etudes et de Recherches pour la Promotion de la Santé, Kangu, Zaire, (no date), 144 pp. In French. This book explains clearly (with good illustrations and diagrams) all aspects of the problems of intestinal parasites and suggests imaginative approaches to the education of the community against worm infestation. Group teaching is highly recommended in the hope of achieving collective community action against these common infections, and detailed instructions for latrine construction are given.

118   van der Heyden, A., Courtejoie, J., Rotsart de Hertaing, I., *Malaria.* Bureau d'Etudes et de Recherches pour la Promotion de la Santé, Kangu, Zaire, 1977, 125 pp. Available in French and English. Designed for health educators to teach the fundamental aspects of malaria, this book gives details of the biology of the malaria parasite and its mosquito host. Included are methods of presenting these facts in association with a series of 62 pictures available as colour slides or posters. Smaller black and white versions of these form a major section of the publication.

119   **Vaughan, A. B.,**
Anaesthetics. The Oxford
Handbooks for Medical
Auxiliaries, Oxford University
Press, London, 1969, 306 pp.
Although based on conditions in
East Africa, this is a book of
great value to three categories of
anaesthetists in all parts of the
world: the fully trained medical
auxiliary; the doctor who is not a
specialist in anaesthetics; and
the untrained auxiliary. For the
latter, there are chapters dealing
with simple, practical
techniques. The book would be
useful both for auxiliaries and
for their teachers. It is clearly
written, very well illustrated
with line drawings and
photographs, and has useful
appendices.

120   **Venezuela, Ministerio de
Sanidad,** *Manual Normativo
para Auxiliares de Enfermeria y
Otro Personal Voluntario
(Training Manual for Auxiliary
Health Workers and Other
Voluntary Personnel).*
Department of Health and
Social Welfare, Caracas, 1971,
212 pp. In Spanish. Health care
services for the rural population
in Venezuela, as in most
developing countries, are either
very poor or nonexistent. This
manual has been developed for a
19-week course to train auxiliary
health workers in an attempt to
improve these services where
they are most needed. It covers
the symptoms and treatment of
most of the common diseases,
methods to improve
environmental sanitation, and
first aid for various types of

injuries. After the course, the
auxiliary workers are sent to
rural health centres where they
receive weekly visits from their
rural zone doctors.

121   **Voluntary Health
Association of India,** *Catalogue
of Educational Materials.*
Voluntary Health Association of
India, New Delhi, 1977, 36 pp.
Intended for all levels of
personnel in rural health and
development programmes and in
hospitals, this catalogue of
low-priced educational materials
describes the pamphlets, charts,
books, film strips, colour-slides
and flash cards for use in health
education in developing
countries. Subjects covered
include child health,
administration and management
of health facilities, anaesthesia
and surgery, nutrition, and
environmental health. Many of
the materials, which are
classified for audience
suitability, are appropriate for
use by auxiliaries and are
available in several Indian
languages.

122   **Voluntary Health
Association of India,** *More about
Child Care.* Voluntary Health
Association of India, New Delhi,
1977, 74 slides, 17 pp. This is a
set of filmstrips/slides focusing
on nutrition. It is intended to
assist health workers to
recognise undernutrition in its
early stages, and to be able to
advise mothers and their
communities how to prevent it. It
has four parts: child care before
birth; diagnosis of

undernutrition; causes of undernutrition; and treatment. Simple and practical advice is given and the set could be useful for training all categories of health workers. Questions for discussion are included after each set. Valuable for adaptation elsewhere.

123 **Voluntary Health Association of India,** *The Training of Traditional Birth Attendants (Dais).* Voluntary Health Association of India, New Delhi, 1977, 30 slides/ 16 pp. This slide-set describes the Integrated Health Services Project of Miraj Medical Centre, Maharashtra, India. The project, which runs a training scheme for traditional birth attendants (*dais*), aims to improve the knowledge of the practising *dais* by giving them regular classes every month. The training has been practical, and *dais* have also been trained to promote health through health education. The *dais* form the necessary link between the people and the health staff. Good description of an important concept in primary health care.

124 **Volunteers in Technical Assistance (VITA),** *Village Technology Handbook.* VITA, Mount Rainier, Maryland, 1975, 400 pp. Also available in Spanish. This well-produced booklet has many excellently prepared line drawings and detailed plans. It covers water resources, health and sanitation, agriculture, food processing and preservation, and home

construction at village level. It is written in simple English and recommended for those concerned with village development.

125 **Wakeford, Richard E.,** *Teaching for Effective Learning—a Short Guide for Teachers of Health Auxiliaries.* REMAHA (Reference Materials for Health Auxiliaries), WHO, Geneva, 1974, 62 pp. This booklet is intended as part of a package to help teachers of health auxiliaries, and is to be used together with selected reference books and a set of illustrations. It aims to give the teacher an understanding of the main principles of teaching and to show how to use these in conjunction with the suggested aids. It also deals with evaluation of both teaching and learning.

126 **Wakeham, Patricia F.,** *Plan for a Village Health Programme Using Village Health Workers.* Emmanuel Hospital Association, New Delhi, 1976, 46 pp. Available from Voluntary Health Association of India, New Delhi. Written for those with the responsibility for developing community health outreach schemes, this definitive plan describes the aims, objectives, strategy, and methods to be used for implementing a programme to bring low-cost health care to villages. It stresses that planning must be positive yet flexible, and gives instructions for programme

evaluation. Appendices cover the responsibilities of key personnel, an outline of a training course for village workers, and a list of drugs and their uses.

127 **Watson, James,** *Pocket Book of Drug Dosages and Procedures for Health Extension Officers.* Para Medical College, Madang, Papua New Guinea, 1974, 194 pp. This pocket book is designed as a 'ready reference' guide for Health Extension Officers in Papua New Guinea who are responsible for rural health centres. The handbook includes information on drug dosages, procedures, and management schemes for specific problems. The maintenance procedures which are essential for proper storage and usage of drugs and equipment are also given. Entries under anaesthetics, contraception, and snakebites and serum tests are particularly useful.

128 **Watt, David G.,** *Emergency Dentistry—Intended for those who must treat the occasional dental patient.* Clausen Publications, Weybridge, U.K., 1975, 65 pp. This illustrated and brief book is intended for those who must treat the occasional dental patient. It covers basic oral anatomy, diagnosis, dental abcesses and other dental infections, emergency treatment of severe facial injuries, anaesthesia, tooth extraction, etc. A useful practical and reference book for auxiliaries and their trainers.

129 **Werner, David,** *Where There Is No Doctor—a Village Health Care Handbook.* The Hesperian Foundation, Palo Alto, California, 1977, 470 pp. Available from TALC (see entry 114). Also available in Spanish, *Donde No Hay Doctor,* (published by Editorial Pax-Mexico). This handbook has been written primarily for those who live far from medical centres, in places where there is no doctor. It explains in simple words and drawings what a villager and health worker can do to prevent, recognise, and treat many common illnesses. It covers a wide range of problems which affect the health of the villager—from diarrhoea to tuberculosis, from helpful and harmful home remedies to the cautious use of certain modern medicines. Special importance is placed on cleanliness, a healthy diet, and vaccination. The book also covers in detail both childbirth and family planning. Very useful for everyone concerned with health care in rural areas.

130 **Wheate, H. W.,** *A Guide to the Teaching of Leprosy in Tanzania.* Ministry of Health and Social Welfare, Dar es Salaam, 1971, 69 pp. Written in fairly technical language, this booklet is designed to make the facts about leprosy available to the non-specialist teacher with a medical or scientific background. It deals in detail

with the background facts about leprosy, its clinical features, treatment and control, and health education. There are student handouts (one in Swahili) throughout the manual, which is illustrated with diagrams and two maps.

131   **White, H. A.**, *Personal Hygiene and Public Health; Health Education; Nursing Arts Notes; Taking a History; Symptomology; Notes on Various Specific Diseases.* Medical Auxiliaries Training School, Sudan Interior Mission, Jos, Nigeria. These materials, which are used in the Medical Auxiliaries Training School, are comprehensive and suitable for senior medical auxiliaries.

132   **Wood, B. S. B.**, *Paediatric Vade Mecum.* Lloyd Luke Ltd., London, 1977, 190 pp. This clear and concise handbook for doctors includes sections on nutrition, the newborn, infections, paediatric emergencies, biochemical information, and paediatric prescribing. Much of the information is tabulated for easy reference. Useful as background material for teachers of auxiliaries but not for auxiliaries themselves.

133   **Wyatt, G. N. and Wyatt, J. L.**, *Medical Assistants' Manual—A Guide to Diagnosis and Treatment.* McGraw Hill, Singapore, 1973, 512 pp. This manual is designed to help the medical assistant in diagnosis and treatment, and contains a useful symptom index. The book emphasizes the prevention of disease and encourages medical assistants to teach their patients the basis of good health. It has a list of drugs and dosages, and is well illustrated.

134   **World Health Organization**, *Guidelines for Evaluating a Training Programme for Health Personnel* by Katz, F. M., WHO Offset Publication No. 38, Geneva, 1978, 35 pp. This concise publication describes one approach to evaluation, by presenting a series of 29 guidelines for the evaluator. The guidelines are organized into four phases: orientation, design of the evaluation, collection of information, and analysis and reporting. Each guideline is a task or action statement, and is accompanied by a brief justification. A set of procedures and necessary additional comments is included. An annex to the guidelines describes a hypothetical example of their use.

135   **World Health Organization,** *Manuel de Normes et Guide Pratique pour les Auxiliaires Infirmiers des Postes de Santé de la Circonscription Sanitaire de Puno (Manual of Standards and Procedures for Nursing Auxiliaries in Health Posts in the Puno Health Area).* By Ortega et al, WHO, Geneva, 1973, 164 pp. This comprehensive manual, now translated into English and

French from the original in Spanish (see entry 88), is intended for rural health workers based in village health posts. Although written for a special region, it contains much material that is suitable for general application by rural health planners and village health auxiliaries. It includes valuable lists, tables and a bibliography.

136 World Health Organization, *Manuel d'Obstétrique à l'Intention des Infirmières de la Santé Publique (Midwifery Manual for Community Health Nurses).* REMAHA, WHO, Geneva, 1974, 223 pp. In French. First written for public health nurses in Papua New Guinea (see entry 84), the latest edition is now available in both French and English. This manual would be useful both for teachers of auxiliary health personnel concerned with midwifery and as a reference book for auxiliaries.

137 World Health Organization, *Manuel de Santé Infantile à l'Intention des Infirmières de la Santé Publique (Child Health Manual for Community Health Nurses).* REMAHA, WHO, Geneva, 1970, 167 pp. In French. First written in Papua New Guinea, and the final edition prepared by David Bowler (see entry 15), this manual has now been translated into French. It is a very useful manual about child health suitable both for teachers of

health auxiliaries and for the use of auxiliaries themselves.

138 World Health Organization, *Manuel Technique de l'Agent Sanitaire Rural (Manual of Procedures for the Rural Health Assistant).* By Gonzales et al. REMAHA, WHO, Geneva, 1972, 117 pp. Also available from UNICEF in UNIPAC. First written in Spanish by a multi-disciplinary group in Costa Rica (see entry 44) and now translated into English and French, this is a very useful all-purpose manual for village health workers especially for reference purposes. It contains useful lists and is clear and comprehensive.

139 World Health Organization, *The Primary Health Worker: Working Guide, Guidelines for Training, Guidelines for Adaptation* (experimental edition). WHO, Geneva, 1977, 338 pp. This book is a revised edition of a WHO working document entitled 'Training and Utilization of Village Health Workers'. It is meant to be adapted to conditions in different countries rather than for use as a definitive manual, and the working guide section is based on the problems that the primary health worker may face during daily work. The guide covers communicable diseases, maternal care, child health, village and home sanitation, common illnesses, and community development. Annexes include medicines, some techniques, anatomical diagrams, an index, and a glossary.

140 **World Health Organization,** *The Training and Utilization of Feldshers in the USSR* (Public Health Paper No. 56). WHO, Geneva, 1974, 52 pp. Details of training and utilization of feldshers in the USSR, where the feldsher system has a remarkable record of health coverage of the rural population, are described. Curricular are included in this useful background reading for anyone interested in the use of various grades of medical auxiliaries.

141 **Zaire, Bureau d'Etudes et de Recherches pour la Promotion de la Santé.** The bureau publishes a series of manuals for nurses and teachers, some of which are reviewed separately in this bibliography. It also produces many materials on health education for nurses, teachers, and students as well as a series of illustrated brochures on many health education aspects including maternal and child health, health education for young people, and preventive measures. Colour slide sets are also available. A complete list of these materials may be obtained from the Bureau, Kangu, Zaire.

142 **Zaire, Centre Protestant d'Editions et de Diffusion (CEDI),** *Enseigne la Santé (Teach Good Health)* by Fountain, D., CEDI, Kinshasa, (no date), 43 pp. In French. The booklet is written for health educators and people in positions to influence others in matters of personal hygiene and preventive health care. For each of ten separate but related subjects it describes in non-technical language why each is a potential health hazard, and suggests simple practical ways of surmounting the problem. Simple illustrations complement the well-written text.

143 **Zambia, Ministry of Health,** *Therapeutics in the Health Centre.* Medical Assistants Training School, Lusaka, 1973, 64 pp. Designed to help registered medical assistants in the use of those drugs available to rural health centres, this book contains some useful tables and an index of medicines.

144 **Zambia, National Food and Nutrition Commission,** *The A B C of Nutrition* by Thomsen, Birtha, The National Food and Nutrition Commission, Lusaka, 1970, 30 pp. This booklet is a guide for teaching nutrition in secondary schools and teacher training colleges in Zambia. Types of malnutrition and their diagnosis and treatment are detailed. The manual emphasizes the need for an increased intake of protein, calcium, iron and vitamins during pregnancy. A glossary of definitions, tables of weights and measures, and several illustrations are included.

Auxiliaries and Community Health and Development

145 **Adams, G. C.,** *Aspects of Technical Education and Training in Africa.* Bulletin of the Aberdeen University African Studies Group (Aberdeen), No. 9, Sept. 1973, pp. 22–39. This article looks into the background, problems and methods of technical education in Africa. It also discusses the recruitment, training, and employment of technical personnel, who are much needed in developing countries.

146 **Ademuwangun, Z. A. and Familusi, J. B.,** *Mother and Child Health in Africa: the Role of Health Education.* Israel Journal of Medical Science (Jerusalem), Vol. 13, No. 5, 1977, pp. 508–515. Presented at the Second Conference on Health Education in Africa, Yaounde, Cameroon, March 23–25, 1976. This paper stresses health education as an important facet of mother and child health services, which should be based on the proper understanding of the needs of the community, and the optimum use of all available facilities, resources and methods of communication. Health education helps to encourage people to participate in the identification of problems and programme planning, and health education projects must approach health problems not only from the individual patient point of view, but from the perspective of the total community.

147 **All Africa Leprosy and Rehabilitation Training Centre (ALERT),** *Essentials of Leprosy.* Edited by Pearson, J. M. H. and Wheate, H. W., ALERT, Addis Ababa, 1977, 64 pp. This booklet is designed for doctors, medical students and senior leprosy workers. It covers treatment of leprosy and its complications, and gives a definition of leprosy, its history, clinical features and classification; notes on anti-leprosy drugs and treatment of the disease are some of the subjects covered in the booklet. Appendices and tables are also included.

148 **All Africa Leprosy and Rehabilitation Training Centre (ALERT),** *Rural Area Supervisors Course: Jan–May 1971. Summary of Sessions on Management.* ALERT, Addis Ababa, (no date). This summary

describes a programme of nine one-hour sessions devised to fit into ALERT's Rural Area Supervisor's Course (see entry 4), to maximise management skills and leadership potential. It should be useful in planning courses for medical auxiliaries who may be responsible for supervising a wide range of less skilled workers.

149   **Alpers, M. et al.,** *Summary Report of the Aboriginal Studies Group, School of Medicine.* University of Western Australia, Shenton Park, Western Australia, 1971, 23 pp. The group undertook a survey during 1970–1971 to obtain a general picture of the medical status, public health needs, community life, and special problems of Aboriginal communities in Western Australia.

150   **Amidi, S.,** *The Effectiveness of Village Health Workers for Primary Health Care in Southern Iran.* Courier of the International Children's Centre (Paris), Vol. 27, No. 2, 1977, pp. 109–112. In Kavar, Southern Iran, 16 villagers were selected for a 6-month course, covering practical sanitation, maternal and child care, treatment of common illnesses, and first aid. They were then posted to villages as auxiliary health workers. Within one year, attendance at the village clinics increased, and infant mortality and birth rates dropped. The programme has been evaluated

and a table of statistics is included.

151   **Andreano, R., Cole-King, S., Katz, F., Rifka, G.,** *Assignment Report: Evaluation of Primary Health Care Projects in Iran.* WHO, Alexandria, June 1976, 44 pp. In 1976, a WHO mission was invited to Iran to evaluate various rural health projects which used minimally trained front-line workers (FLWs). They interviewed personnel, examined records, and calculated the cost of implementing this type of programme at national level. The team recommended that a method of constant feedback be used in order to gauge the effectiveness of the proposed national programme.

152   **Bangladesh, Gonashasthaya Kendra,** *Progress Report Number 4.* Gonashasthaya Kendra, District Dacca, 1974, 10 pp. This document reports on the working of the programme which covers 13 sub-centres and uses about 23 paramedics, more than half of whom are women. The family planning campaign has been particularly successful because paramedics and volunteers provide advice and the contraceptive pill to women at home. The centre also runs a health insurance scheme, and vocational training for women. A scheme for agricultural improvement using 'para-agros' is being prepared.

153 **Bangladesh,
Gonashasthaya Kendra,** *Progress
Report Number 6.*
Gonashasthaya Kendra, District
Dacca, Dec. 1977, 12 pp. The
6th progress report of the
Gonashasthaya Kendra,
comments on the improved
status of women through the
activities of the project, and
covers the progress of the
Kendra in agriculture,
agricultural loans, vocational
training, education, family
planning, and health.

154 **Bayoumi, A.,** *Medical
Auxiliaries in Family Health—
Some Ideas and Examples.*
Paper delivered at the 4th
International Conference of the
Sudan Association of
Paediatricians, Port Sudan,
February 15–18, 1975, 8 pp.
This paper discusses why the
Sudanese health care system has
failed to reach the majority of
the population in rural areas,
and the attitudes that perpetuate
the present system. By
comparing hospital-based with
community-based health care,
and curative with preventive and
promotive care, the paper makes
valuable suggestions for the
redefinition of the role of
professionals, and advocates
greater emphasis on the training
of auxiliaries.

155 **Bayoumi, A.,** *Primary
Health Care: An
Epidemiological Approach.*
Paper delivered at the 2nd
International Congress, World
Federation of Public Health
Associations and the 69th
Annual Conference, Canadian
Public Health Association,
Halifax, Canada, 23–26 May,
1978, 14 pp. The development of
an epidemiological model for
primary health care represents
one of the most challenging tasks
in reforming the general health
care delivery system in recent
times. A new approach to the
prevailing traditional system of
clinical diagnosis and treatment
is one which provides an
epidemiological framework
within which issues of primary
health care can be examined.
Methods of epidemiological
analysis for community
diagnosis can in turn help to
design community health action
programmes. Useful example of
innovative thinking.

156 **Bayoumi, A.,** *The
Training and Activity of Village
Midwives in the Sudan.* Tropical
Doctor, (London) Vol. 6, July
1976, pp. 118–125. The article
shows the dramatic growth in
the training of midwives in the
Sudan. Numbers trained per
year increased from 10–38 at the
first training school in Omduran
in 1921, to a total of 523 at 16
schools, each in a provincial
headquarters, in 1975. The
article describes the course and
practical training received by
traditional midwives from areas
all over the country, selected for
maximum geographical
coverage, with priority given to
areas in critical need of
midwifery services. The 9
months training covers antenatal
care, child welfare, home
visiting, general hygiene, normal

and complicated pregnancy, and the use of simple drugs.

157 **Behrhorst, C.,** *Programme Description: Chimaltenango Development Programme.* Presented at the International Medical and Research Foundation Symposium on the Community Health Worker, Warrenton, Virginia, 26–28 October, 1977, 11 pp. The Chimaltenango programme in Guatemala is an integrated and comprehensive project which works in all aspects of community development, with emphasis on community involvement. Committees drawn from local communities consider their needs in social, economic, and health fields. The programme uses agricultural extension workers (AEWs) and rural health promotors (RHPs). The RHPs' training emphasizes symptom treatment and recognition of common illnesses, using a simple manual. The AEWs are also local men and women trained in preventive medicine as well as in agriculture.

158 **Blumhagen, Rex V. and Blumhagen, J.,** *Family Health Care: A Rural Health Care Delivery Scheme—Final Report with Summary of Experiences and Recommendations for a Health Care Delivery System.* Medical Assistance Programmes (MAP), Illinois, U.S.A., 1974, 105 pp. This report is based on 6 years' experience of the Medical Assistance Programme in the U.S.A. In the first 2 years mobile clinics were held, and the next 4 years were spent on operating a base hospital and health centre. This report sets out the information and experience gained from these projects. A bibliography, samples of questionnaires, forms used in data collection, lists of tables, charts, a map, and abbreviations are included.

159 **Bollag, U.,** *Is the Community Health Aide in Jamaica Well Prepared for the Detection of Protein-energy-malnutrition?* Courier of the International Children's Centre (Paris), Vol. 27, No. 4, 1977, pp. 338–346. In Jamaica, in a young children's nutrition programme, community health aides use weight-for-age charts which are based on the Harvard standards, rather than on readily available local data. The weight-for-age charts are useful for assessing growth, but are inadequate for detecting malnutrition unless other data, such as anthropometric measurements, are also available. The author feels that community health aides should concentrate on giving necessary nutrition education.

160 **Bomgaars, R.,** *Shanta Bhawan Community Health Services 1975 Report.* Shanta Bhawan Hospital, Kathmandu, Nepal, 1975, 10 pp. The report describes the community health services of the Shanta Bhawan Hospital located in the southern part of the Kathmandu Valley of

Nepal, which involves 22 villages. The report covers such areas as community participation, seminars and training sessions, and the production of educational and training materials.

161   Bonsi, S. K., *Persistence and Change in Traditional Medical Practice in Ghana.* International Journal of Contemporary Sociology (Ghaziabad), Vol. 14, Nos. 1 & 2, 1977, pp. 27–38. Most traditional healers are anxious to learn new ideas, methods and herbal practices, as data from a sample of 150 healers in Southern Ghana shows. At the Institute of Traditional Medicine, healers can learn the preservation and administration of herbal preparations, and the use of some Western medical technology. This is important from the community health point of view, as traditional healers can lay the foundations within the local established system for the standardization of medical practice. Some references are included.

162   Borus, J. F., *Neighbourhood Health Centres as Providers of Primary Mental Health Care.* The New England Journal of Medicine (Boston), Vol. 295, No. 3, July 15, 1976, pp. 140–145. The article reports on 19 Boston neighbourhood health centres which have mental health programmes as part of their primary health care system. They provide indirect consultative services to general health staff, who refer forty-eight per cent of the centres' patients. Children constitute forty-three per cent of these patients, and twenty-two per cent of services are outreach visits, primarily to patients' homes. Such neighbourhood centres increase the accessibility and psychological acceptability of mental health services and enhance case finding, successful referral, and coordination of primary health care.

163   Browne, S. G., *The Role of the Rural Dispensary in Combating an Epidemic of Poliomyelitis.* The National Fund for Research into Crippling Diseases, London, 1965, pp. 9–16. Although written in 1965, this paper (which is printed in French and English side by side) is still a very useful document. Early diagnosis of poliomyelitis is vitally important so that proper treatment can be initiated and measures taken to limit the spread of the disease. The well-trained medical auxiliary can cope with both the acute and the rehabilitation stages.

164   Browne, S. G., *Vocational Rehabilitation of Leprosy Patients in Africa.* Available from ILO, Geneva, Ref. ILO/TAP/AFR/RII, 1969, pp. 73–78. The present improved outlook for leprosy means that patients and ex-patients should, given the right kind of help, be able to support themselves satisfactorily within the community to which they belong.

165 **Browne, S. G.,** *Training of Medical Auxiliaries in the Former Belgian Congo.* The Lancet (London), No. 7812, 19 May 1973, pp. 1103–1105. This article discusses a programme for medical auxiliaries in the former Belgian Congo (Zaire). It describes the programme's admission requirements, curricula, teaching staff, examinations, and other activities. Nine references are listed.

166 **Browne, S. G.,** *The Diagnosis and Management of Early Leprosy.* The Leprosy Mission, London, 1975, 36 pp. This booklet, written mainly for medical practitioners, contains practical advice on the recognition and treatment of early leprosy. A series of colour photographs show the early symptoms of tuberculoid, borderline, and lepromatous leprosy, and the section on treatment discusses useful drugs, dosages, and reactions. Useful for trainers of auxiliaries.

167 **Bryant, John,** *Health and the Developing World.* Cornell University Press, London/New York, 1969, 333 pp. Health problems in Africa, Latin America and Asia are examined and solutions are suggested, with special attention given to manpower needs. Useful background material for planners of public health programmes.

168 **Bryant, John,** *Community Health Care (review).* In Christian Medical Commission Annual Meeting 1971, Geneva, pp. 67–69. The author maintains that there are three types of health care system. The first, a hospital, deals with a few people, all seen by a doctor. The second, a comprehensive community health centre, deals with more people, seen by auxiliaries. In the third type, with community involvement, the doctor acts as manager, consultant and leader, reducing his role as decision-maker. The second type becomes the third when the community becomes aware and is willing to take the responsibility for decision-making.

169 **Butt, H. W.,** *Nutrition Programmes for Children: Suggestions to Implement a Practical Programme.* Indo-Dutch Project for Child Welfare, Hyderabad, India, 1975, 16 pp. The Indo-Dutch Project for Child Welfare initiated a scheme giving free meals to malnourished children in Hyderabad, which was not successful. Therefore, in order to improve education and health services, auxiliary nurses and teachers were approached to persuade the villagers to participate in the scheme. Farmers were encouraged to produce the correct components for a protein supplement, as a result of which 7,000 children are now no longer malnourished.

170 **Byrne, Kathy,** *The Health Promoter, Department of Olancho, Honduras, Central America: Programme Description.* El Programma de Promotoras de Salud, Olancho, Honduras, May 1976, 42 pp. An important system of rural health care, using village women in campesino homemakers' clubs in Olancho to eradicate the diseases common in rural Honduras, is described. The health workers are volunteers who are trained in simple curative and preventive medicine in three months. Their chief functions are to educate women in the clubs, to keep records, to give primary health care, and to dispense medicines. Diagrams and appendices are included.

171 **Callan, Lawrence B.,** *Supervision, the Key to Success with Aides.* Public Health Reports (Washington), Vol. 85, No. 9, Sept. 1970, pp. 780–787. This article discusses the essential concepts of supervision, techniques of applying them, and their results. The author emphasizes the need to invite aides into the decision-making process to break the hierarchy of health personnel. To assist supervisors in evaluating their own performance, a comprehensive list of questions about their practices is given. A selected bibliography is also included. Very useful.

172 **Canada, Department of National Health and Welfare,** *Methods Manual for Community Health Workers.*
Department of National Health and Welfare, Ottawa, 1970, 30 pp. Also available in French. This manual describes in simple terms techniques of community organization and the fundamentals of group and communication dynamics. It covers communication, interviewing, working with committees, groups and local government. It also includes modern educational and social change theory.

173 **Canada, Department of National Health and Welfare,** *The Community Health Worker in Indian and Eskimo Communities.* Department of National Health and Welfare, Ottawa, (no date), 9 pp. This document describes the selection and training programmes of community health workers in Indian and Eskimo communities of Canada, and their relationship with public nurses. It also gives their job description and emphasizes the need to give them inservice training, as well as to include them in professional discussions, in order to raise their confidence in the performance of their duties. Good background material for teachers.

174 **Canadian Universities Service Overseas (CUSO),** *Readings in Health.* Canadian Universities Service Overseas, Ottawa, 1973, 355 pp. This large, well-chosen collection of articles reprinted from local newspapers, medical journals, textbooks, etc., is intended as an

aid to orientation for Canadian volunteer health workers. It includes sections on nutrition, maternal and child health, family planning, education and training, and projects. Interesting background material which gives a world-wide view of developments in health care.

175   **Carlaw, Raymond W.,** *Development of Interaction as an Approach to Training.* Public Health Reports (Washington), Vol. 85, No. 9, Sept. 1970, pp. 754–759. The techniques of training used in the South Pacific are outlined, with emphasis on the interaction between the trainee, the community, and the trainer. The author suggests that all training must relate to the trainee's past experience. The article covers the preparation of a training programme, its implementation, and the post-training feedback. It includes a discussion of the learning process.

176   **Centre International de l'Enfance,** *Comparative Analysis of the Retrospective Studies of Growth and Development in Venezuela* by de Limongi, I. P. et al. Presented at XIIeme Réunion des Equipes Chargées des Etudes sur la Croissance et le Developpement de l'Enfant Normal, Centre International de l'Enfance, Paris, Dec. 1974, 11 pp. This analysis of studies on the growth and development of Venezuelan, Peruvian, and Mexican children concludes that important differences in size and weight exist according to social class. Venezuelan children appear to mature earlier than British children, and between the ages of 8 and 11 they are practically as tall as British children of the Tanner standards.

177   **Chabot, H. T. J.,** *The Chinese System of Health Care: An Inquiry into Public Health in the People's Republic of China.* Tropical and Geographical Medicine (Amsterdam), 28, 1976, pp. S88–S134. This review covers a wide range of subjects; a description of health services and manpower in pre-revolution China, the development of the present system, aspects of Chinese communist philosophy which have been vital to the new approach to health, the influence of traditional philosophy, and the extent to which the Chinese experience is applicable to health services elsewhere. References included.

178   **Chen, P. C.,** *Medical Auxiliary in Rural Malaysia.* The Lancet (London), No. 7810, 5 May 1973, pp. 983–985. In order to reduce rural poverty and ill health in Malaysia, steps have been taken to establish a health service with a series of health centres and a staffing system which relies mainly on auxiliary health workers. Local midwives are given training in simple hygiene, and included in the health programme. Further planning includes the retraining of midwives in child health, and also the training of assistant nurses in midwifery for their

roles as community
nurse-midwives.

179   **Christian Medical
Commission,** *Contact.* Christian
Medical Commission, Geneva.
This paper, produced by the
Commission about 6 times a
year, usually contains one article
per issue, some of which are
translated into French or
Spanish. The articles are
frequently on rural health care
and community health projects
in developing countries, and
each issue has a notes section
which gives details of new
publications, films, etc.

180   **Christian Medical
Commission,** *Community Health
and the United Mission to Nepal
(UMN).* Christian Medical
Commission, Geneva, 1972. The
Christian Hospital at Tansen
plans to train 136 village health
volunteers in a 2-week
programme of physiology,
hygiene, common diseases,
sanitation, nutrition, and first
aid. After returning to work in
their own areas, they will be
visited every three months by
UMN-employed, trained
medical auxiliaries acting as
supervisors. The importance of
health education and the need to
provide suitable material for
health teaching at village level
are stressed. Materials should
include information on
agricultural extension work and
family planning.

181   **Christian Medical
Commission,** *Health Care in
China: an introduction.*

Christian Medical Commission,
Geneva, 1974, 140 pp. Also
available from TALC (see entry
114). What is a 'barefoot
doctor'? How did the Chinese
rid their country of venereal
diseases? What are the Chinese
doing about birth control? These
and many other questions are the
subject of investigations by a
study group in Hong Kong. In
this report they discuss how the
Chinese in the People's Republic
have organized health services to
provide care for 800 million
people. The purpose of this book
is to stimulate those concerned
with health care elsewhere in the
search for solutions to pressing
health care needs. Useful
background reading and a very
useful annotated bibliography.

182   **Christian Medical
Commission,** *Kojedo
Community Health Project.*
Christian Medical Commission,
Geneva, 1972, 12 pp. This report
describes the development of a
community-centred health
programme on a South Korean
island, which has recognised the
need to train auxiliaries to
maintain a village network of
primary health care and health
education.

183   **Christian Medical
Commission,** *Review of Health
Services in Botswana with
particular reference to Mission
Medical Services.* Christian
Medical Commission, Geneva,
1972, 44 pp. Surveyors of
Botswana's health services found
that mission medical services
would have to integrate with

government services for survival. This would require adjustments, as missions' understanding of administrative practices or health economics was minimal. It is recommended that missions establish a central administration among themselves. Descriptions of church-related medical institutions are given, a syllabus for the family welfare educators' course is summarised, and a scheme for training medical auxiliaries is appended.

184 **Ciba Foundation,** *Teamwork for World Health.* Edited by Wolstenholme, G. E. W. and O'Connor, M., Churchill Livingstone, Edinburgh, 1971, 242 pp. Available from the Ciba Foundation, London. In a collection of 16 papers at a symposium on Teamwork for World Health, seven papers deal specifically with health care in developing countries and especially with development and use of auxiliary health workers. A bibliography on rural health care is included.

185 **Commonwealth Foundation and National Fund for Research into Crippling Diseases,** *Disabled in Developing Countries.* Commonwealth Foundation, London, 1977, 148 pp. Proceedings of a symposium on Appropriate Technology and Delivery of Health and Welfare Services for the Disabled, Oxford, 26–30 September, 1976. This report contains 25 papers, most of which are concerned with the physical and mental rehabilitation of the handicapped. They cover the manufacture and improvisation of aids, management and treatment of the disabled, care of leprosy and poliomyelitis patients, and care of handicapped children. There are some papers on planning of health care delivery in developing countries. Discussion on each paper, and conclusions and resolutions arising from the conference are also included.

186 **Community Systems Foundation,** *Nutrition Planning—An International Journal of Abstracts in Food and Nutrition Planning.* Community Systems Foundation, Ann Arbor, Michigan, U.S.A. This journal is published quarterly and it contains about 20 documents covering agriculture; food processing; public and curative health; nutrition education; social, cultural and religious influences on nutrition; comprehensive programmes etc. Useful for trainers who want to keep in touch with the latest developments in different areas of the world in these subjects.

187 **Conde, Julien,** *Some Demographic Aspects of Human Resources in Africa: Three background papers prepared for the expert working group meeting held in Dakar, February–March 1973.* OECD Development Centre, Paris, 1973, 236 pp. Two of these three papers cover the effects of changes in fertility and mortality

on the socioeconomic structures of African populations, and the effect of the development of health services on mortality in Africa. The third paper includes detailed case studies of four African countries that illustrate approaches to planning of human resources, including the use of medical assistants.

188   Correa, H., *Measured Influence of Nutrition on Socio-Economic Development.* World Review of Nutrition and Dietetics (Basel), Vol. 20, 1975, pp. 1–48. This paper gives the methods used and the results obtained in studying the impact of nutritional conditions on socioeconomic development. It shows their effect on physical and mental capacities, educational achievement, and productivity. Though a fairly academic and technical paper, it could be useful background material for training institutes and for teachers.

189   D'Aeth, R. G., *Memorandum on Health Planning in Lesotho based on St. James Mission Hospital, Mants'oyane.* St. James Hospital, Mants'oyane, Lesotho, 1974, 19 pp. The use of medical auxiliaries and rural health centres could extend the area covered by the services of the St. James Hospital. A 10-year plan proposes the building of 11 health centres, each to be staffed by two staff nurses and two nurse-aids. A further two to four aides would be located in surrounding villages to advise

the local community on nutrition and hygiene. The 'Flying Doctor Service', already in operation, is a necessary part of the service. Appendices to the memorandum provide a comprehensive breakdown of the costs of the plan.

190   Degremont, A. A., Geigy, R., Streibel, H. P., *The Mangoky Project,* Journal of the World Medical Association, International Co-operation in Medicine (London), (no date), pp. 65–69. This article reports on a highly successful project in the control and prevention of schistosomiasis in a 'controlled' area of 2,500 hectares of cultivated land in the valley of the Mangoky River in Southwest Malagasy. It outlines the drugs, dosages and treatments used. Interesting and useful.

191   Development Centre of the Organization for Economic Co-operation and Development, *An Assessment of Family Planning Programmes: Summary Proceedings of the Fourth Annual Population Conference of the Development Centre.* Organization for Economic Co-operation and Development (OECD), Paris, 1972, 195 pp. The volume consists of conference presentations and discussions on the assessment of national family planning programmes. In addition, it covers issues such as administrative structures, field workers, targets, population policies, framework for evaluation, etc. Country by country population data, selected demographic, social and economic indices, and achievements of government-sponsored family planning programmes are also included.

192   **Dickson, A.**, *Youth's Contribution to Health Care: Paediatrics in Reverse?* Commonwealth Secretariat, London, 1975, 30 pp. The author argues that voluntary youth workers, if trained, could make considerable contributions to health care in the developing countries by learning the rudiments of diagnosis, treatment, and prevention of some of the more common ailments within their own communities. At a more advanced level, medical school applicants could be trained as health auxiliaries, or could work within their own communities, before being accepted by medical schools.

193   **Dunnill, Peter,** *Provision of Pharmaceuticals by Appropriate Technology.* Appropriate Technology (London), Vol. 4, No. 2, August 1977, pp. 16–17. The author feels that drugs can be produced locally if pharmaceutical auxiliaries are trained in their formulation, packaging and storage. This would reduce the cost of pharmaceutical imports. Greater savings could be made if the government controlled the range of drugs used, imported from the cheapest supplier, and supported other appropriate

technologies such as packaging, storage and stock recycling methods.

194   **East-West Communication Institute,** *Report on the Inter-Regional Seminar-Cum-Workshop on the Integrated Use of Folk Media and Mass Media in Family Planning Communication Programmes. New Delhi, India, October 7–16, 1974.* East-West Communication Institute, Honolulu, Hawaii, 1975, 16 pp. Abstracts of papers presented at the seminar-cum-workshop, which discussed the integration of folk media into communication programmes, are presented. The seminar showed the methods by which folk media have been mobilised to promote family planning in India. These abstracts include papers on folk forms in different areas of India, and their adaptation for use by the mass media in family planning communication. Useful.

195   **Ebrahim, G. J.,** *A Model of Integrated Community Health Care —Community Health Care in a Rural Area.* Tropical and Geographical Medicine (Amsterdam), Vol. 28, 1976, pp. S5–S52. This paper surveys the provision of health services in developing countries in the context of development: the urban/rural maldistribution, demographic patterns, resources, social structures and organization. The paper suggests a model of integrated community health care

including curative, preventive and promotive activities which provides regular health supervision, communicable diseases control, nutrition programmes, family planning services, clean water etc. A list of references is included.

196 **Edwards, P. J.**, *Teaching Specialist English: with special reference to English for nurses and midwives in Nigeria.* English Language Teaching Journal (Oxford), Vol. 28, No. 3, April 1974, pp. 247–252. This article describes the teaching of English to medical students for whom English is a second language. The students need a foundation vocabulary to understand the lectures, and to be able to recognise medical terms in speech, and to make them proficient in note-taking and summarising, etc. Beyond this stage, instruction should become increasingly responsive to the problems of each individual student.

197 **Elliott, Katherine,** *Meeting World Health Needs: The Doctor and the Medical Auxiliary.* World Hospitals (Oxford), July 1973, pp. 94–97. Reprinted in World Medical Journal (London), Vol. 23, No. 3, 1976, pp. 42–45. The author discusses the limitations of world health care due to a shortage of doctors and lack of funds. 80% of people in developing countries live in rural areas, but 80% of doctors are to be found in the urban areas. The solution seems to lie in the use of medical auxiliaries, who could be trained in a very short period to perform routine medical functions. Support and encouragement from professionals is essential, and administrators must take a lead in providing and working with auxiliary health teams.

198 **Elliott, K.**, *Year of the Health Auxiliary?* In British Health Care Planning and Technology: Year Book of the British Hospitals Export Council, London, 1975, pp. 79–87. Many countries are now using health auxiliaries who have been trained, not as substandard doctors, but as the most relevant people to give primary and preventive health care at village level and health education in their own communities. Health workers should also have some knowledge of agriculture and industry in order to help their communities to overcome the problems of poverty and disease.

199 **Engler, Tomas A.,** *An Evaluation Scheme for Polyvalent Health Assistants in a Rural Area of the Republic of Panama.* Hospital de Changuinola, Bocas del Toro, Panama, (no date), 9 pp. The paper summarises a programme in Bocas del Toro, where health assistants were trained to improve the health of the population through education, community organization, and the provision of minimal primary medical care. It also gives a multi-method design for the evaluation of the efficiency of

45

health assistants, but the evaluation itself is not included.

200 Essex, B. J. and Everett, V. J., *Use of an Action-orientated Record Card for Antenatal Screening.* Tropical Doctor, (London), Vol. 7, 1977, pp. 134–138. This article reports on a study that was carried out to design and test an antenatal record card which would detect women at risk, indicate the appropriate action for each abnormality, emphasize the treatment needed to prevent anaemia, malaria, neonatal tetanus, and malnutrition, and also provide a record of the outcome of labour. The study was conducted in Dar es Salaam, and outlines data such as risk factors found in the total population, relationship between height, stillbirth, and neonatal death, etc. Very useful article.

201 Fendall, N. R. E., *Auxiliaries in Health Care: Programs in Developing Countries.* John Hopkins Press, Baltimore, Maryland, 1972, 200 pp. Also available in French and Spanish. This book provides information on the need for auxiliary personnel, their potential availability, the possibilities for training them, and their successful utilization. It is intended for use by health planners and administrators, qualified practitioners, and teachers and supervisors of auxiliaries. Various categories of auxiliaries are defined, their functions and training are

discussed, and a suggested curriculum for medical assistants is included. A very useful book.

202 Feuerstein, Marie Thérèse, *Rural Health Problems in Developing Countries: The Need for a Comprehensive Approach.* Community Development Journal (London), Vol. 11, No. 1, 1976, pp. 38–52. This useful paper argues for a comprehensive approach to community health, based on experiences of people working in various countries. It stresses the need to include community health in overall community development. Well written and comprehensive.

203 Fonaroff, Arlene, *Cultural Perceptions and Nutritional Disorders: A Jamaican Study.* Bulletin of the Pan American Health Organization (Washington), Vol. IX, No. 3, 1975, pp. 112–123. An enquiry into the understanding of protein-calorie malnutrition by Jamaican women concluded that, in order to be effective, health education should incorporate new practices into traditional patterns. From interviews it was evident that the traditional treatment of marasmus needed only a change of diet to be successful. Therefore, health educators should aim to modify rather than to change traditional customs.

204 Food and Agriculture Organization (FAO), *Training for Agriculture and Rural*

Development. FAO, Rome, 1975, 147 pp. This annual review of current opinions and experience in agricultural education and extension and their contribution to rural development contains many interesting reports from several countries. It could be very useful for community health programmes using auxiliaries, who are becoming increasingly involved in rural development. The review covers education, inservice training, rural extension services, communications, intermediate technologies, functional literacy, etc.

205   **Food and Agriculture Organization (FAO),** *Equipment Related to the Domestic Functions of Food Preparation, Handling and Storage.* FAO, Rome, 1974. This folder contains detailed descriptions and drawings of how villagers can be helped to develop their techniques of preparing, handling, and storing food in order to maximise nutritional benefit and minimise food wastage.

206   **Fountain, Daniel E.,** *Programme of Rural Public Health, Vanga Hospital, Republic of Zaire.* Contact 13, Christian Medical Commission, Geneva, Feb. 1973, pp. 2–14. This report of a public health project in Zaire describes the various programmes undertaken in 80 villages to improve community health. Programmes include rural sanitation via

health education, family health through monthly family health clinics, malaria treatment, and nutrition education. Village leaders have been successfully involved in the programmes, and a genuine desire for better health has developed among the people.

207   **Ghana, Ministry of Health,** *A Primary Health Care Concept for Ghana.* Ministry of Health, National Health Planning Unit, Accra, September 1977, 36 pp. This is a proposal designed to extend health services to 80% of all Ghanaians by 1990 and to prevent and treat 80% of the disease problems afflicting them. It is based on the premise that health service activities are a part of total social and economic development with the complete involvement of the people at the community level. It covers the description and implementation of the proposed primary health care system, and useful information is appended.

208   **Gideon, H.,** *How much of a hospital's work could be done by paramedical workers?* Christian Medical Commission, Geneva, 1973, 7 pp. This analysis of 1032 outpatients and 681 inpatients from eight mission hospitals in six states in India shows that 48% of outpatients and 44% of inpatients would probably not have needed hospital treatment had they been advised earlier by a paramedical worker. Very useful background material.

209 **Gish, O.,** *Health Planning for Women and Children.* Institute of Development Studies, University of Sussex, Brighton, U.K., 1974, 14 pp. Since mothers and children comprise a large proportion of the population in developing countries, it is important that there is an improvement in mother and child health services. For this, a decentralized system, as in Tanzania, would be appropriate, and more auxiliaries and health assistants should be trained. Active participation of the community, as in China, is essential to ensure that antenatal, maternity, and postnatal care is made available at rural health centres to the majority of the people.

210 **Gish, O.,** *Doctor Auxiliaries in Tanzania.* The Lancet (London), 2 Dec. 1973, pp. 1251–1254. In this article the role of the auxiliary in Tanzania's health services since independence in 1961 is examined. Recognizing that self-reliance in the health sector could not be realised through a system that regarded registered doctors as its sole medical practitioners, Tanzania decided to use its existing auxiliary framework of assistant medical officers, medical assistants, and rural medical aides. A network of health centres and dispensaries to serve the rural population is planned to become effective by 1980, staffed and directed by auxiliaries. A table illustrates recent changes in the workload of health personnel, and the

importance of providing the medical auxiliary with opportunities for continued education is emphasized.

211 **Golden, G. N.,** *Tuberculosis of Bones and Joints.* Mission Hospital Bulletin No. 40, The Medical Missionary Association, London, Feb. 1972, 22 pp. This bulletin explains the pathology, clinical features, diagnosis, general management, techniques of operation, and post-operative treatment of TB abcesses and sinuses in skeletal tuberculosis. It gives further instructions for specific areas such as hips, knees and spinal tuberculosis. Useful for a fairly high level of health worker.

212 **Haire, Doris and Haire, John,** *The Nurse's Contribution to Successful Breast-Feeding.* The International Childbirth Education Association Inc., New Jersey, 1974, 68 pp. This reference material for those working in the field of maternal care in the United States emphasizes sympathetic guidance from the nurse to encourage the mother's breastfeeding. Detailed instructions on how to breastfeed and a description of how the breast functions are given. A checklist is included, in which some of the reasons for a mother's concern appear alongside the causes of the problems, and remedies are suggested.

213 **Haraldson, S.,** *Health Planning in Sparsely Populated*

Areas: With Particular Reference to Mobile Populations of Developing Countries. Department of Social Medicine, Scandinavian School of Public Health, Gothenburg, Sweden, 1973, 39 pp. This pamphlet brings together conclusions and recommendations for health planning based on the author's 20 years of field experience with scattered and nomadic peoples. He advocates a policy of 'guided nomadism', which accepts nomadism as a lifestyle and recognises that planning must occur on a regional basis with use of auxiliaries within a framework of socioeconomic development.

214 **Harinasuta, Chamlong,** *The Need for Clinical Assistants in Thailand.* The Lancet (London), 9 June 1973, pp. 1298–1300. This short article describes the need to train clinical assistants, paramedicals, and medical auxiliaries in order to fill the gap in the Thai health services, particularly in rural areas. It outlines the measures which were taken by the Thai Government to meet this need. Useful article.

215 **Harrison, Paul,** *Basic Health Delivery in the Third World.* New Scientist (London), Vol. 73, No. 1039, 17 Feb. 1977, pp. 411–413. This article reports on two basic health projects in Latin America, one in Colombia and the other in Peru, that use health promoters and simplified medicine for health care in the villages and slums. The author describes the work and limitations of the health promotor, whose functions include first aid, midwifery, vaccinations, taking blood and sputum samples, sanitation, nutrition education, etc. Useful for all personnel working in community health programmes.

216 *Health Education Index.* B. Edsall and Co., London, last edition May 1976. This index, produced approximately every 18 months, is a compilation of available health education materials including all types of visual aids. It contains contact addresses and information sources in the U.K. for a wide range of health problems.

217 **Heese, H. de V.** et al., *Health Care of Children. The Potential Role of the Paediatric Nurse Associate.* South African Medical Journal (Cape Town), No. 48, 1974, pp. 1752–1758. This document is a preliminary report on a training scheme introduced for Paediatric Nurse Associates, which covers their function, qualification, training programme, method of instruction, and evaluation. Paediatric Nurse Associates are a response to the crying need for medical attention, whether it be professional or non-professional, due to the growth of the population, particularly in the 'homelands'.

218 **Heggenhougen, H. K. and Diamond, S.,** *Relevance of Traditional Medicine.* Institut Penyelidikan Perubatan,

International Centre for Medical Research, University of California, Kuala Lumpur, November 1976, 36 pp. Presented at the Atlanta Symposium of the Albert Schweitzer Centenary, Atlanta, 7 April 1975. The authors suggest that the understanding of traditional medicine is important for the planning of health programmes, and conclude with a description of the Behrhorst Health Development Programme that includes positive elements of Western and traditional practice. The programme was established in 1962 and serves 200,000 Cakchiquel Indians by using health promoters who orient their work to the social and cultural realities of their people.

219   **Hellberg, J. H.,** *Community Health and the Church.* World Council of Churches, Geneva, 1971, 74 pp. Also available in French. This booklet discusses the appropriate use of available resources to make health services accessible to the great majority of people. It covers topics such as nutrition, sanitation, steps toward community health, the use of auxiliaries, weight charts, data gathering, etc., and is not solely concerned with church-related medical work. A reading list is included.

220   **Hesperian Foundation,** *Project Piaxtla and the Hesperian Foundation.* The Hesperian Foundation, Palo Alto, California, (no date), 5 pp. This is a brief report of the campesino-run health care network that covers several thousand square miles of mountain terrain and serves a population of more than 10,000 persons living in 100 small settlements. Project Piaxtla attempts to involve the mountain communities in a process of meeting their own health needs in a manner that is economically realistic, ecologically sound, and personally humane. The project emphasizes preventive medicine and health education. The most important activity is the training of village health workers or promotores de salud.

221   **Hendrata, L.,** *A Model for Community Health Care in Rural Java.* Department of Service and Development, Council of Churches in Indonesia, Jakarta Pusat, Indonesia, Jan. 1975, 15 pp. This well written paper discusses the evolution of a health centre into a community health care programme by the people using health cadres and a village health insurance scheme. This model is remarkable for its originality and simplicity, as it has grown out of the day-to-day grappling with actual problems in the community, together with the people of the community. A short bibliography is included. Very useful.

222   **Hendrickse, R. G.,** *Technologies for Rural Development—Provision of Basic Paediatric Care.* Liverpool

50

School of Tropical Medicine, University of Liverpool, U.K., 1976, 15 pp. This paper is concerned with the redistribution of medical resources based on the essential needs of people. It stresses that the medical requirements of children should be provided in rural community hospitals, and covers the most important health problems of the developing countries. Appropriate health methods and techniques are indicated. Useful background material.

223 Hobdell, M. H., *Suggestions for the Organization and Teaching of a Tanzanian School of Dentistry, University of Dar es Salaam.* Department of Community Dentistry, London Hospital, London, (no date), 10 pp. To make dental education relevant to the health needs and resources of people in developing countries, the author emphasizes the need to integrate academic, social, economic and political factors into the curriculum, and to make dentistry part of a health team effort. The paper includes: designing a curriculum model, dental schools and field service centres, integration of dental and auxiliary personnel training. A very useful document on dentistry.

224 Hoff, Wilbur, *The Importance of Training for Effective Performance.* Public Health Reports (Washington), Vol. 85, No. 9, 1971, pp. 760–766. This article stresses the need for suitable training of auxiliaries in the United States to cover such topics as communication, identifying health problems, and general administrative duties. Training should also recognise desirable skills and knowledge, use appropriate teaching methods, etc. The importance of evaluation is emphasized, and a selected annotated bibliography on health aides is included.

225 Howlett, G. Gordon, *Using Projectors Away from Mains Electricity* Educational Development. This article could be of great value to people involved in health education in remote parts of their country, where electricity supplies are not available. The article describes various methods of converting/adapting conventional equipment to work on batteries or other supplies. Very useful.

226 Hsu, Robert S., *The Barefoot Doctors of the People's Republic of China—Some Problems.* New England Journal of Medicine (Boston), Vol. 291, No. 3, July 1974, pp. 124–168. The article discusses the disadvantages of the system of barefoot doctors and stresses that it should not necessarily be accepted as a model to emulate. It suggests that 'barefoot doctors' should be thought of as a stopgap measure and that the Chinese system may need modification if it is to be usefully copied elsewhere.

227   **Hubbard, Charles,** *Como Orientar en Planificación Familiar (How to Organize Family Planning).* Translated from 'Family Planning Education', C. V. Mosby Co., St. Louis, U.S.A., 1975, 250 pp. In Spanish. This book describes the anatomy and physiology of reproduction and contains a complete description of methods for birth control with relative merits and drawbacks, including sterilization and abortion. It also discusses venereal disease. Useful for doctors, nurses, and other medical personnel.

228   **Hudson, H. E. and Parker, E. B.,** *Medical Communication in Alaska by Satellite.* New England Journal of Medicine (Boston), 30 Dec. 1974. This article describes an important experiment to use a highly technological 'back-up' method to support village health auxiliaries with a minimum of training, who have to work in considerable isolation in Alaska.

229   **Indo-Dutch Urban Project for Child Welfare,** *Abstracts of Research on the Health Component.* Indo-Dutch Urban Project for Child Welfare, Hyderabad, India, 1976, 48 pp. These abstracts cover a wide range of subjects in social medicine, especially in the areas of paediatrics, maternal and child health, nutrition, etc., with particular emphasis on an integrated approach to community health. They include annotations of 32 studies on planning supplementary feeding with local cereals, evaluating growth patterns of children from 6–36 months, and the effect of selected weaning schemes on the growth pattern of infants below the age of 3 years. Useful.

230   **Indo-Dutch Urban Project for Child Welfare,** *Fighting Malnutrition with 'Hyderabad Mix'.* Indo-Dutch Urban Project for Child Welfare, Hyderabad, India, (no date), 6 pp. This pamphlet describes the use of local ingredients for making protein packs for the prevention of malnutrition in developing countries. The protein pack, the recipe for which is given, can be prepared by mothers in India using the available foods in villages.

231   **Indo-Dutch Urban Project for Child Welfare,** *Model Balwadi-Cum-Field Training Unit, Chevella.* Indo-Dutch Urban project for Child Welfare, Hyderabad, India, 1976, 6 pp. The role of 'Mother-Teachers', or mothers from rural areas who are trained as pre-school teachers, is described. These mothers practise nutritional health education in the communities. The programme, which covers 12 balwadis (pre-schools), proves that rural Indian women can play an active role in development by being involved in the activities of health and nutrition education. Useful.

232   **Intermediate Technology Publications Ltd.** Intermediate Technology Publications

distributes and publishes the largest collection of publications on intermediate technology which cover many aspects of community development, such as agriculture and fish culture, building, cooperatives, health, industrial business and management, methane, rural workshops, social economics, sourcebooks, water, wind power, etc. Titles of interest in health include *Health Manpower and the Medical Auxiliary; How to Make Basic Hospital Equipment; Gardening for Better Nutrition,* etc. A complete publications list can be obtained from Intermediate Technology Publications Ltd., London.

233 **International Secretariat for Volunteer Service,** *The Mobilization of Response Structures from the Grassroots towards Health Services: Report on a Workshop.* International Secretariat for Volunteer Service, Asian Regional Office, Manila, 8–11 July 1974, 128 pp. This report of a workshop held in Manila contains descriptions of some of the most successful community health projects in many parts of the world, including Sri Lanka, India, Bangladesh, Indonesia, the Western Pacific region and others. Also included are papers on community participation in community health programmes.

234 **Ivory Coast,** *Hôpital Protestant de Dabou.* Dabou, Ivory Coast, 1972, 12 pp. This document describes the operation since 1968 of the hospital's 3-year course for training local people to provide high quality nursing care in small hospitals and mobile clinics. Plans for health education courses, a rural maternity training centre, and a nutrition/antenatal village project are discussed. Appendices include the nurse training curriculum, a report of the mobile clinic work, and a resume of projected expansion.

235 **Jagdish, V.,** *Reorganization of Health Auxiliaries in India.* School of Hygiene and Public Health, Department of International Health, John Hopkins University, Baltimore, Maryland, Aug. 1976, 8 pp. This paper reviews the services of auxiliaries in primary health care in India. It outlines the staffing of a primary health care centre and shows the need for, and the evolution of, multi-purpose workers, supported by health workers. Useful for those interested in understanding the structure of primary health care in India.

236 **Jamaica Council for the Handicapped,** *Proceedings of the Caribbean Regional Conference on the Handicapped Child.* The Caribbean Institute on Mental Retardation and Developmental Disabilities, Kingston, 1975, 171 pp. This Regional Conference on the 'Handicapped Child' emphasizes the need for comprehensive planning and the use of non-professionals, trained in basic skills, to assist in the

preventive and curative care of communities. Papers and discussions cover early detection and diagnosis of handicaps, alternative strategies for intervention, special education programmes, etc. May be useful as background information for trainers and planners of auxiliary programmes.

237 **Janssens, P. G., Why** *Medical Auxiliaries in the Tropics? Lessons of a Meaningful Past.* Bulletin of the New York Academy of Medicine (New York), Vol. 48, No. 10, Nov. 1972, pp. 1304–1313. This article, which describes the origin and development of medical auxiliary training programmes in Zaire, gives examples of successful implementation, training drawbacks, and opposition to such schemes. The author believes that in order to strengthen the basic health services it is imperative to upgrade the educational programme of the low and middle-level auxiliaries within the limits of technical and vocational training. Training should be according to national health priorities based on family and community needs, not according to international standards.

238 **Jayatilaka, A. D.,** *Sarvodaya and Delivery of Health Care in Sri Lanka.* In 'Mobilisation of Response Structures from the Grassroots towards Health Services: Report of a Workshop', International

Secretariat for Volunteer Service, Asian Regional Office, Manila, 8–11 July 1974, pp. 46–55. The Sarvodaya Shramadana Sangamaya, which began in Sri Lanka in 1958 as a community development movement based on Buddhist philosophy, is described. 70% of the population in Sri Lanka presently depend on the services of traditional ayurvedic practitioners, who could be trained with volunteer Sarvodaya workers in primary health care and disease control. This would help to meet the major health needs of the rural population.

239 **Jelliffe, Derrick B. and Jelliffe, E. F. Patrice,** *Dyadic Nature of Mother and Child Nutrition.* UNICEF, Carnets de l'Enfance-Assignment Children (Geneva), No. 35, July–Sept 1976, pp. 104–110. Summaries in French and Spanish. The recognition of infant feeding as a biological dyadic phenomenon not only gives better insight, but also permits a rational, feasible and low-cost approach to mother-child nutrition in developing countries. This article covers maternal nutrition and the weaning period, and contrasts patterns of nutrition in rich and poor communities.

240 **Jelliffe, E. F. Patrice,** *A New Look at Multimixes for the Caribbean,* Journal of Tropical Pediatrics and Environmental Child Health, Vol. 17, 1971, pp. 136–150. This detailed article shows the need and the methods

required for providing adequate mixed diets for adults, children and infants in all communities. It gives the nutritive values of various foods, in order to make it easier for trainers and auxiliaries to understand the value of multimixes. Useful background material for teachers and auxiliaries involved in community nutrition projects.

241 Johnson, Anne M., *Health Services and Socio-Economic Development in Venezuela.* School of Medicine, University of Newcastle, U.K., March 1975, 31 pp. This is a realistic view of the health services in Venezuela in the context of socioeconomic development. It points out that if the marginal urban poor and the isolated rural poor are to be covered by the Health Services, a rethinking is required, and more auxiliaries instead of doctors must be trained. The efforts of coordination that various Government Departments have made to achieve better health standards for these sections of the population are given by the author. A bibliography is included.

242 Johnson, Anne M., *Integrated Health Services— The Panamanian Experience.* School of Medicine, University of Newcastle, U.K., June–Sept. 1976, 18 pp. A study of the community health facilities provided by the Integrated Health Services (IHS) of a province in Panama is reported. This reveals that poor

communications and disruption of indigenous culture have been obstacles to the IHS, which is presently overstaffed with doctors who are reluctant to join health teams. Auxiliaries, who are responsible for primary health care, community organization, environmental health, and health education in the area's isolated communities, are attempting to mobilise local health committees.

243 Joseph, Stephen C., *The Health Care Team Demonstration: An Experiment in Rural Health Training for Nursing and Medical Students in Central Africa.* Presented at the 8th annual meeting of leaders of Macy-supported Paediatric Programs in Latin America and the Caribbean, Brasilia, Brazil, 4 Feb. 1974, 15 pp. This paper describes an experiment involving a multi-disciplinary approach in the teaching of medical personnel by exposing them to a rural health centre setting and to the experience of functioning as a team to analyse problems in community health. The paper shows the deficiencies of such a programme which may be of use to others contemplating similar teaching methods in other countries. A list of references is also included in this most useful paper.

244 Joseph, Stephen C., *Protein-calorie Malnutrition in West African Children.* Rocky Mountain Medical Journal (Denver), July 1974, Vol. 71,

No. 7, pp. 403–405. This useful article describes the symptoms and causes of nutritional deficiency, such as marasmus, protein-calorie malnutrition and kwashiorkor. The author feels that the starvation problem is world-wide, and that malnutrition will continue to be a major cause of child mortality in the foreseeable future. This short paper compares the different types of malnutrition which often relate to the specific diets of people. A list of references is included.

245 **Joseph, Stephen C.**, *The United States and Health in the Developing Countries: Alternatives for Action.* Commission on Critical Choices for Americans, Nov. 1974, 72 pp. This general view of global major health problems critically and comprehensively discusses the current trends and crucial problems of health in the developing countries. It covers the causes, prevention, cures, and economic factors involved in eradicating major diseases and syndromes such as pneumonia, diarrhoea, hookworm, trachoma, schistosomiasis, tuberculosis, malaria, leprosy, etc. Includes many useful tables and an extensive list of references.

246 **Kagimba, J.**, *Community Based Maternal and Child Health/Family Planning Educator: A Key Person in the Chogoria Community Health Project.* International Medical and Research Foundation, Warrenton, Virginia, U.S.A.,

1977, 6 pp. A community health project established in 1973 by Chogoria Hospital, Kenya, which aimed to provide a network of rural dispensaries, home visiting, immunization, and delivery of family planning services, involved the training of maternal and child health/ family planning educators. The health educators are women from the village who are trained in the theory and practical methods of family planning, child care, and communication techniques. As a result of the programme, the number of family planning acceptors has increased considerably.

247 **Karlin, Barry P. H.**, *The State of the Art Study—A Report on 180 Health Projects in 54 Countries.* Salubritas (Washington), Vol. 1, No. 1, Jan. 1977, pp. 1–5. Paper delivered at the Mexican Society of Public Health, Cancun, Mexico, 26 Oct. 1976. This paper introduces some of the data collected from 180 health projects in 54 countries; in Africa, Asia and Latin America. It explains the utilization of manpower and the delivery of health services including family planning, nutrition, and health education. The planning, management and evaluation of these projects are also covered. The study may be useful background information for planners and teachers.

248 **Khuri-Otaqui, S.**, *Family Service Centre Programme— Description and Analysis.* Near

East Ecumenical Committee for Palestine Refugees, Nicosia, Cyprus. Also available from the Christian Medical Commission, 1972, 54 pp. Following the 1948 conflict in the Middle East, the Near East Council of Churches Committee for Refugee Work promoted a series of programmes to provide Palestinian refugees with food, shelter and clothing. By 1963 a number of centres were established along the West Bank, the Gaza strip, East Jordan and in the Lebanon. The most important purpose of the centres was educational; community development was integrated; self-help emphasized. Home visits were essential and auxiliary workers were trained and used as widely as possible. Staff were given inservice training.

249 **Komaroff, A. L.** et al., *Protocols for Physician Assistants.* New England Journal of Medicine (Boston), Vol. 290, No. 6, pp. 307–312, Feb. 1974. This article concludes that health assistants can successfully care for patients, after brief training only, provided that protocols are available for their guidance. The limits of their competence must be clearly indicated within the protocol, which should not be too rigid. The system works particularly well in dealing with conditions such as hypertension and diabetes, which require constant supervision, but not always necessarily the attention of a physician.

250 **Koppert, Joan,** *Nutrition Rehabilitation—Its Practical Application.* Tri-Med Books Ltd., London, 1977, 130 pp. This down-to-earth book dealing with the planning and organization of nutrition rehabilitation programmes covers topics such as financing, staff selection, diets, record-keeping and evaluation. It emphasizes the involvement of mothers in the programme, as they can transfer good nutrition and health ideas to the community. Very useful for workers involved in maternal child health, health education, and community development programmes. Well illustrated, and references included.

251 **Korea, Seoul National University,** *Chunseong Gun Community Health Programme.* School of Public Health, Seoul National University, Seoul, Korea, July 1975, 130 pp. This programme, established in Korea in 1972, aims to provide field training to improve the health care services to the rural population, and to set up a model community health programme. Mothers' clubs have been started to recruit local women to act as primary health workers. The paper has many tables of facts and figures, and is most useful for any group wanting to establish a community health programme.

252 **Kumar, S.,** *Information and Documentation Needs for Health and Family Welfare Professionals.* National Institute of Health and Family Welfare,

New Delhi, November 1977, 15 pp. The National Institute of Health and Family Welfare in India is creating a new National Documentation Centre to collect, process, analyse, and disseminate practical health-related information from various institutions, libraries, etc. in the country. Services to be provided by the Centre include an abstracting bulletin, bibliographies, document copying, a technical enquiry system, and translation facilities to make information from abroad available to users. A list of addresses of organizations in S.E. Asia concerned with health and family welfare is included.

253 **The Lancet.** Published weekly, this journal contains occasional articles on the use and training of auxiliaries in health care. A series of articles in 1973–74 (the 'Medical Alliance' series) included such titles as:
Health Care Extension using Medical Auxiliaries in Guatemala by E. Croft Long and Alberto Viau, Vol. 1, p. 127, 26 Jan. 1974.
Is the Chinese 'Barefoot Doctor' exportable to rural Iran? by H. A. Ronaghy and S. Solter, Vol. 1, p. 1331, 29 June 1974. Other titles in the series are annotated separately in this bibliography.

254 **Larsson, U. and Larsson, Y.,** *Child Health in Developing Countries—The Role of the Expatriate Doctor.* World Medical Journal, (New York), Vol. 21, No. 2, March–April

1974, pp. 36–38. This description of the work of paediatricians and mother and child health workers in a Swedish development assistance programme since 1959 stresses the need for the physician to teach and to delegate. The training of auxiliary health personnel is of paramount importance for the success of all assistance programmes.

255 **Laugesen, Murray,** *Better Care in Leprosy.* Voluntary Health Association of India, New Delhi, 1978, 64 pp. Written in simplified English and illustrated with black and white and colour photographs, cartoons, and line drawings, this excellent booklet explains the cause, diagnosis, and treatment of leprosy. It is meant for village health workers, teachers, and social workers, who are encouraged to show the book to adults and children in the villages. The need to spread knowledge about leprosy and to refute superstitions about the social and clinical aspects of the disease is stressed throughout.

256 **Lawrence, D., Wilson, W. M. and Castle, C. H.,** *Employment of MEDEX Graduates and Trainees—Five Year Progress Report for the United States.* Journal of American Medical Association (Chicago), Vol. 234, No. 2, 1975, pp. 174–177. The MEDEX approach to the training and deployment of physician extenders is described and contrasted with other

physician-extender training models, and results of a survey of 277 MEDEX graduates and 207 trainees are presented. Practically all MEDEX graduates and trainees are employed in the rural areas of the United States, which suggests that the strategy used to place MEDEX practitioners into communities requiring additional health services has been successful.

257 **Lee, George E.** et al., *Labrador Community Health Project.* Memorial University of Newfoundland Extension Service, Canada, Nov. 1974, 8 pp. This paper describes a pilot project to produce a health education programme relevant to the needs of specific communities living in the coastal area of Labrador. The extension service also has a working paper (1975) about adult education programming throughout the province.

258 **Leiliabadi, G. A.** et al., *Project for Health Services Development Research in Iran: Coverage of personal health care needs through frontline health workers in selected areas of West Azerbaijan.* Iranian Public Health Association/ International Epidemiological Association Meeting, Isfahan, 8–11 March 1976, 14 pp. This paper describes the provision of health care services for the underserved rural population by new frontline health workers, selected from the community. After a short period of training

they can contribute to the improvement of personal health, maternal and child health, family planning. The general background and implementation of the project, which serves a population of 130,000 in 300 villages, are described. The selection and methods of training of these frontline workers is given, and references are included.

259 **Lesotho, Ministry of Health and Social Welfare,** *Village Health Worker in Lesotho: A Report of a Workshop held on 26–27 March 1977 at Tsakholo Health Centre.* Ministry of Health and Social Welfare, Maseru, Lesotho, Aug. 1977, 77 pp. This report, which consists of four chapters and twelve appendices, contains a tabulated comparision of three ongoing village health worker (VHW) programmes in Lesotho at the Quthing, Scott and Tellebong hospitals. It gives summaries of the workshop's three sessions, which cover the job description of the VHW, implementation of the VHW programmes at village level, development of the organizational framework for a VHW programme, and recommendations for future programme development.

260 **Levitt, Sophie,** *Helping the Handicapped Child at Village Level* In 'The Disabled in Developing Countries', Commonwealth Foundation, London, 1977, pp. 47–50. The paper suggests that there may be

simple methods of devising exercises for the disabled child's primary development that can be initiated by parents, teachers, or health workers at home, in schools or in the wider community. Also, one person per village could be trained to advise and instruct in this field, backed possibily by a mobile specialist.

261   **Lolik, P. L.** et al. *Primary Health Care Programme in the Southern Region of the Sudan.* Presented at the International Medical and Research Foundation Symposium on the Community Health Worker, Warrenton, Virginia, U.S.A., 26–28 October, 1977, 13 pp. This paper reports on the Primary Health Care Programme for the Sudan, which aims to train community health workers (CHWs) during a 9-month practical course. This course aims to qualify the CHW to assist the village midwife, advise on maternal and child health care, control communicable diseases, recognize common causes of sickness, give appropriate treatment, and keep records. The CHW has charge of a Primary Health Care unit and is supervised by the Medical Assistant.

262   **Lutheran World Service,** *Village Technology Handbook.* Lutheran World Service, Geneva, 1977, 366 pp. Also available from Rural Communication Services, South Petherton, U.K. This looseleaf folder compiles names and addresses in many countries of organizations, people, and projects involved in any aspect of rural development, with special emphasis on appropriate methods and technologies. Its objective is to make new ideas and techniques available to a larger audience. The folder includes addresses of contact groups and persons listed by country, international organisations, and a list of books and periodicals. Useful for many levels of interest in a rapidly expanding field.

263   **Mabry, E. G.,** *Planning a Community Health Programme.* Christian Medical Association of India, Nagpur, 1972, 56 pp. Also available from TALC (see entry 114). Church-related hospitals in Indian communities should increasingly be involved in community health activities outside the confines of the hospitals. The book provides guidelines for the redeployment of mission hospital staff according to objectives which are modest and clearly set out. If fulfilled, a good basis would be established on which more extensive and ambitious community health programmes could be established. This is a unique document which has a great contribution to make to Community Health.

264   **Mager, Robert and Beach, Kenneth,** *Education of Instructors in Vocational Training.* Fearon Publications, Palo Alto, California, (no date), 120 pp. Also available in

60

Spanish. This is very useful for designing effective teaching methods for various vocational on-the-job and formal and informal training.

265 **Mahler, H.**, *Health—A Demystification of Medical Technology.* The Lancet (London), Vol. 2, No. 7940, 1 Nov. 1975, pp. 829–833. This paper describes how the mystique of medical technology and the traditional hierarchical attitudes of the medical profession prevent the provision of medical care for the majority of people as early, cheaply, and acceptably as possible. It advocates the delegation of responsibility for health care from physicians to nurses and mothers, to provide better coverage by health services without loss of quality.

266 **Mata, L. J., Kromal, R. A., Urrutia, J. J. and Garcia, B.,** *Effect of Infection on Food Intake and the Nutritional State: Perspectives as Viewed from the Village.* American Journal of Clinical Nutrition (Bethesda), Vol. 30, No. 8, Aug. 1977 pp. 1215–1227. A study in Guatemala between 1964 and 1972 on food intake, morbidity, and intestinal infections in a group of 45 village children aged 0–3 years, revealed that infection in young children caused extremely high morbidity, particularly during the weaning period. Infections such as diarrhoea were important causes of weight loss, impaired physical growth, severe malnutrition, and death. An important health aspect for inclusion in the training of health workers.

267 **Mata, L. J.,** *Antenatal Events and Postnatal Growth and Survival of Children— Prospective Observation in a Rural Guatemalan Village.* In 'Proceedings Western Hemisphere Nutrition Congress IV,' White, P. L. & Selvey, N., eds., Publishing Sciences Group, Inc., Acton, Massachusetts, 1975, pp. 107–116. This technical paper, which may be of use to trainers of higher levels of auxiliaries, summarises observations of a long-term field study in a typical Indian village in the Guatemalan highlands. 203 women and 465 pregnancies were observed for birth interval, midpregnancy weight, height, obstetrical experience and socioeconomic conditions, etc. Illustrated with tables and graphs. References are included.

268 **McCallister, Theissen and McDermott,** *Hacia Mejores Programas de Planificación Familiar.* C. V. Mosby and Co., St. Louis, U.S.A., 1975, 432 pp. Translated from *Readings in Family Planning: A Challenge to the Health Professions.* C. V. Mosby and Co. Discusses particularly the problem of inadequate personnel. This is an excellent book discussing many aspects of family planning medical care and contains three special articles written by Latin American specialists in the field.

269   McDowell, J., *Village Technology in Eastern Africa* UNICEF Eastern Africa Regional Office, Nairobi, 1976, 63 pp. UNICEF sponsored Regional Seminar on Simple Technology for the Rural Family, Nairobi, 14–19 June, 1976. This book, which reports on the development and extension of technologies that are appropriate to rural villages in Eastern Africa and other developing countries, is intended as a reference source. It covers basic concepts and UNICEF policy, social aspects of appropriate technology, energy, food production, conservation and preservation, and water supplies. Health aspects are also included, and a detailed description of a village technolgy unit designed to implement and demonstrate appropriate technologies is given.

270   McDowell, J., *Kayunga Nutrition Scouts Project: An Outline of a Successful Nutritional Surveillance/ Prevention Project in Uganda.* UNICEF, Nairobi, Sept. 1977, 6 pp. This is a report of a successful community-supported, low-cost nutritional surveillance and prevention project, using teenage scouts at Kayunga in Uganda. Twelve of these scouts, selected by the community and trained for six weeks, cover about 400 households. The scouts advise mothers on nutrition, child care and domestic sanitation. The project has aroused community interest, and a water supply and sanitation programme are envisaged in the future.

271   Mehra, S., *Pre-testing of 'Better Child Care' booklet.* Voluntary Health Association of India, New Delhi, 1977, 15 pp. 'Better Child Care', a booklet to be used by village health workers, was pre-tested in the States of Gujarat, Tamil Nadu, and Uttar Pradesh in India. The objective of the pre-test was to assess village people's understanding of photographs to be used in the booklet, and to assess the readability of the text. Appropriate methodology was designed to make it possible for village health workers to carry out the test. The tabulation of results and the methods used has been outlined. (See also entry 72).

272   Mellander, O., *Nutrition and Health Care in Preschool Children—A Report from China.* Medicinsk-Kemiska Institutionen, Goteborg Universitet, Goteborg, Sweden, 1972, 23 pp. This report is based on a 3-week study tour in April 1972 to medical schools, paediatric departments, general hospitals, and health centres in Peking, Shanghai, and Canton and rural communes outside the cities. Useful background reading, especially in relation to nutrition.

273   Morley, David, *Paediatric Priorities in the Developing World.* Butterworths Postgraduate Paediatrics Series, Sevenoaks, U.K., 1973, 470 pp.

Also available from TALC (see entry 114). In examining the problems facing child health services in the developing world, this book emphasizes the social, economic, cultural and ethical considerations which are often ignored by most medical schools. Specific conditions like diarrhoea, acute respiratory infections, measles, whooping cough, malaria, tuberculosis and anaemia are comprehensively described. A chapter on the objectives and running of under-fives clinics is included, and the book also covers record systems, communication, management, and nursing. Many sections are suitable for senior medical assistants and other health workers. Invaluable background material for anyone involved in planning auxiliary training courses at any level.

274 **Mwabulambo, D. J.,** *Village Health Workers Scheme in Tanzania.* Presented at the International Medical and Research Foundation Symposium on the Community Health Worker, Warrenton, Virginia, 26–28 Oct. 1977, 7 pp. Village posts manned by village medical helpers (VMHs) were introduced in Tanzania in 1969 to provide health care in areas previously without any health facilities. VMHs, who are selected by the community, undergo 3 months training at the district hospital, then return to work in the village on a voluntary basis. The responsibilities of the VMH include running the village

health post, treating minor ailments, and increasing local awareness of the importance of preventive medicine. There are now VMHs in 2,020 villages and by 1980 about 5,600 villages will benefit from their services.

275 **Myers, S. E.,** *Operating Dental Auxiliaries.* WHO Chronicle (Geneva), Vol. 26, No. 11, Nov. 1972, pp. 511–515. The article discusses the activities of dental auxiliaries throughout the world, and some recent training programmes for them in Uganda, Senegal, Papua New Guinea, etc. The number of operating dental auxiliaries, the number of training centres, and the estimated number of students have been documented in two tables according to country.

276 **Nchinda, T. C.,** *An Integrated Approach to the Training of Health Personnel for Developing Countries: the Cameroon Experiment.* Tropical Doctor (London), Vol. 1, Jan. 1974, pp. 41–45. The activities of the University Health Sciences Centre at Yaounde in the Cameroons are described. This is a unique experiment where all members of the health profession are trained as a team. This method assists each of the workers to understand each other's function and also to learn to work as a team. The outcome of this experiment will be significant for the pattern of health care in this area of the world.

63

277 **Neumann, A. K.** et al., *The Role of the Indigenous Medicine Practitioner in Two Areas of India.* Social Science and Medicine Journals Dept., New York, Vol. 5, 1971, pp. 137–149. Interviews with 72 rural indigenous practitioners in two districts of India are reported, as well as the result of observation of their work diagnosing and treating 542 patients. The training of the indigenous practitioners varied from a few months apprenticeship to 6 years formal training in recognised schools of medicine. They outnumber modern (allopathic) practitioners by 10:1, and are well regarded by the villagers. The report suggests more studies should be carried out on this subject as indigenous practitioners could play an important role in community health services.

278 **Nordberg, Olle; Phillips, Peter; Sterky, Göran,** Eds., *Action for Children: Towards an Optimum Child Care Package in Africa.* The Dag Hammarskjöld Foundation, Uppsala, 1975, 238 pp. This book contains progressive ideas and views by sociologists, social workers and educationists on the African situation with special reference to children. It covers many important areas of child health, such as the early years of the child, child and society, perinatal care, nutrition, immunisation, with cost effective studies and a package for delivering services. Many

references and interesting illustrations included.

279 **Nugroho, Gunawan,** *Dana Sehat An Experiment in Raising Community Health Standards in Solo (Central Java): Community Health Insurance Scheme.* Panti Walujo Hospital, Solo, Indonesia, 1972, 20 pp. Describes a simple, practical and cheap method of raising health standards in two small communities in Indonesia. It involves a community health insurance scheme based on mutual cooperation, and presents health in a wide context of community development. This simple system could be used as a framework for both curative and preventive health care depending on the conditions and situations in the community. A very useful concept that may be of value for experimentation elsewhere.

280 **Nugroho, Gunawan,** *Community Participation in a Community Health Programme and Community Health Insurance.* In 'Mobilisation of Response Structures from the Grassroots towards Health Services: Report of a Workshop', International Secretariat for Volunteer Service, Manila, 8–11 July 1974, pp. 105–112. The author emphasizes that local people should be involved at all stages of a community health programme. The paper reports on two successful projects in Java. The first, in Solo, runs an insurance scheme set up by the local people, and is self-supporting. The other

project, in Sirkandi, is also financed by the local community. Both projects mainly cover environmental health, but also include some major agricultural and sanitary innovations.

281 Nutrition Rehabilitation Centre, *Project Proposal to Indian Council of Medical Research—The Village Health Worker Programme.* Nutrition Rehabilitation Centre, Government Erskine Hospital, Madurai, India, 1977, 13 pp. This proposal describes a community health programme which started in 1973 as a rural nutrition education programme and now intends to cover the entire block of Thiruppuvanam, Ramnad District, Tamil Nadu in South India. At present the project covers about 30 of the 43 panchayat villages in the block. The proposal includes the objectives and development of the programme, and a description of the project area. The project description covers village health committees, selection of VHWs, training, referral, coverage, etc.

282 Nyirenda, F. K., *Under Five Clinics: Normal/Underweight Children.* League for International Food Education Newsletter (Washington), Feb. 1978, pp. 3–4. In Malawi, normal and underweight children are divided at an under-fives clinic, so that undernourished children can receive the special attention they require. This helps to assist mothers with underweight children in the necessary health education, and special care for immunization, which is not always as effective in undernourished children.

283 O'Donnell, Michael, *Who Knows Best What Patients Need?* World Medicine (London), March 21 1973, 6 pp. This project, headed by Dr. Wirjawan of the Indonesian Ministry of Health, trains nurse-tutors. Adopting national dress, the nurses work in the villages to discover what people want. When they have done so, they persuade the villagers to provide money, labour and materials to help meet their own needs. The nurses then become neighbours, seeking advice from their teachers; acting for the people to bring health services to a receptive community. It is hoped that by training these nurses to teach others, they can build a health system rooted in the community.

284 Office of Health Economics, *Medical Care in Developing Countries.* Office of Health Economics, London, U.K., No. 44, Nov. 1972, 40 pp. With the urgent necessity in the developing countries for the prevention and the treatment of malnutrition; communicable diseases; the promotion of family planning, and sanitation— hospitals and medical education have proved expensive and unproductive. Auxiliary health workers can provide efficient primary care, but they need suitable training and an adequate system of referral and guidance. This booklet mentions auxiliaries already practising in many parts of the world and recognises the widespread introduction of auxiliaries as essential for adequate rural coverage.

285 **O'Keefe, M.**, *Evaluation of Medical Missions, A Pilot Report.* Christian Medical Commission, Geneva, 1973, 6 pp. This pilot study analyses the community health needs rather than hospital statistics, in order to evaluate the effectiveness of Zambian medical missions. It shows that hospitals may meet the needs of the individual, but the needs of the community go unheeded. A useful introduction to methods of assessment.

286 **Ostergard, Donald R.** *Manuel de Gineco-Obstectricia.* Editorial Pax-Mexico, Mexico, 1975, 200 pp. Translated from *Women's Health Care Specialist Training Program Syllabus and Manual,* Harbor General Hospital, Torrance, California, U.S.A. Covers standard obstetrical, gynaecological and physical medical procedures, and typical treatment for non-gynaecological and gynaecological abnormalities, including VD. The procedures and management of complications during pregnancy and also birth control methods are discussed. The manual contains information on lactation, nutrition,

communication in family planning etc. Valuable for doctors, medical aides, interns and nurses, to which the publication is chiefly addressed.

287 **Ozigi, Yusuf O.**, *The Importance of Health and Nutrition Education in the Training of Rural Health Workers in the Northern States of Nigeria.* A special report submitted to the Queen Elizabeth College, University of London, 1976, 82 pp. This unpublished study outlines the role, training and duties of the Rural Health worker. It also discusses the techniques of health and nutrition education and emphasizes the importance of health and nutrition education in the training of rural health workers. Very useful for planners and also for trainers of auxiliaries. A syllabus and bibliography are included.

288 **Pan American Gazette,** *Teamwork for Better Dental Care.* Pan American Gazette (Washington DC), Vol. 5, No. 2, April–June 1973, 3 pp. The article reports on the shortage of dentists in developing countries and suggests that one immediate solution lies in training a large cadre of intermediate-level and auxiliary personnel to help out with the secondary tasks of dentistry. An interesting appraisal of the potential for delegation to auxiliary personnel within a special health field.

289 **Pan American Health Organization (PAHO),** *The*

Delivery of Primary Care by Medical Auxiliaries: Techniques of Utilisation and Analysis of Benefits Achieved in Some Rural Villages in Guatemala. In 'Medical Auxiliaries', PAHO Scientific Publication No. 278 (Washington DC), 1973, pp. 24–37. The use of non-professional personnel to deliver primary medical care in rural areas is described for four different programmes. For comparative purposes two other rural programmes are also presented, where physicians provide the primary care. Measures of coverage, case loads, referral rates and costs are presented. The data given indicate that infant mortality can be halved by use of medical services provided by non-professionals. A useful paper.

290 Papua New Guinea, Department of Public Health, *Papua New Guinea Health Plan.* Department of Public Health, Konedobu, Papua New Guinea, 1974. This comprehensive report outlines the 5-year national health plan for Papua New Guinea which aims to provide basic health services for the entire population. It reviews family health, nutrition, laboratory services, environmental health, the resources available to meet national goals to control major diseases, and a health education programme. Management development, pharmaceutical services, and community involvement are also reviewed.

Many tables and other data are included.

291 Parker, Alberta W., *Health Technology at the Primary Care Level: Working Paper No. 1.* Prepared for a WHO informal consultation on Health Technology, Geneva, 9–12 Feb. 1976, 42 pp. Written as a background document for discussion on health technology, this paper stresses the need to mobilise resources within the community in order to balance health care needs with health care resources. The paper comprehensively covers the alternatives which are available and the need to develop health technology which is effective, simple, acceptable and provided at little cost. Useful for health and project planners of primary health care.

292 Paton, T. J., *A Scheme for Training medical Auxiliaries.* In McGilvray, J. C. and Simmons, G., 'Review of Health Services in Botswana with Particular Reference to Mission Medical Services', Christian Medical Commission, Geneva, 1972, Appendix II, ii–v. This is a report of a small rural health project which trained auxiliary health workers in Botswana. Women were given a 6-week course in first aid, health education, antenatal care, immunization and the recognition and treatment of many common ailments. A list of drugs which could safely be administered by these women was drawn up. The results proved satisfactory—attendance at children's and antenatal clinics improved. Highly recommends the training of more auxiliaries.

293 **Pene, P.**, *Health Auxiliaries in Francophone Africa*, The Lancet (London) Vol. 1, No. 7811, 12 May 1973, pp. 1047–1048. There has always been a scarcity of health workers in Francophone Africa, and therefore many states used auxiliary health workers, but these are beginning to disappear. The number of medical assistants practising in 1973 was estimated to be around 300, with about 10,000 auxiliary nurses who, with a minimum of training could be posted to rural areas as assistants to doctors. Priority should be given to training auxiliary midwives and technicians to work in mobile health units.

294 **Phatak, A. T.**, *Community Health—Our Present Day Problems and Needs*. Paper presented at Second All India Meeting of Medico Friend Circle, Sewagram, India, 27–29 Dec. 1975, 10 pp. This article outlines the health problems of India, the inadequacy of the present system, and the attitudes of medical personnel to meet these needs. The author recommends giving priority to the training of paramedicals and auxiliaries, and coordinating the efforts of those in the various fields of rural development to use available resources to the full in the interests of the entire community. Useful.

295 **Pitcairn, D. M. and Flahault, D.**, *The Medical Assistant: An Intermediate Level of Health Care Personnel.* World Health Organization, Geneva, 1974, 171 pp. Discussions on the use of medical assistants are reported in these proceedings of a 1973 international conference. The medical assistants are health technicians who have received 8–9 years of general education followed by 2–3 years of technical training. The advantages and disadvantages of this level of auxiliary health personnel are considered cross-culturally. The aim of the conference was to extend the possible role of the medical assistant in the improvement of health services, and his/her potential contribution in community development is emphasized.

296 **Pongspipat, Soonthara,** *Auxiliary Health Worker Training in Thailand*. Paper prepared for the 'Asian Seminar on Village Health Worker', Shiraz, Iran, March 1976. Chonburi Health Training Centre, Division of Health Training, Ministry of Public Health, Bangkok, March 1976, 15 pp. The government of Thailand has been training various categories of auxiliaries and paramedicals, such as junior health workers, midwives, dental auxiliaries, laboratory assistants, etc. The paper covers the

problems of auxiliary health worker training and utilization, and the future plans of government to train village health volunteers. It also includes the functions and training curricula for different categories of auxiliary health workers.

297　**Pongspipat, Soonthara,** *Training and Utilization of Village Volunteers in Thailand.* Prepared for the 'Asian Seminar on Village Health Worker', Shiraz, Iran, March 1976. Chonburi Health Training Centre, Division of Health Training, Ministry of Public Health, Bangkok, March 1976, 5 pp. The paper reports on a pilot study in Korat Province during the past six years, using a health communicator, and a village health volunteer, who were responsible for collecting and disseminating health information, disease surveillance, simple medical care, and acting as coordinators between government officials and the villagers. Useful.

298　**Population Crisis Committee and the Victor Bostrom Fund Committee,** *Population and Family Planning in the People's Republic of China.* Edited by Pistrow, P. T., Population Crisis Committee, Washington, 1971, 36 pp. This interesting collection of articles describes the state of family planning in China in 1971. Useful for comparison with later figures which show how much can be achieved in a short time

using a large number of auxiliary health care personnel to reach the community.

299　**Prince Leopold Institute of Tropical Medicine,** *Disaster Epidemiology: Proceedings of an International Colloquium.* Prince Leopold Institute of Tropical Medicine, Antwerp, Belgium, 1976, 219 pp. This is a collection of papers followed by discussions on many aspects of epidemiology and communicable diseases in disaster situations. Various methods are given for the surveillance and prediction of food shortages and malnutrition. Methods of intervention and details of efforts made in some disasters are described, and bibliographies are included.

300　**Quinn, J. R.** (Editor), *China: Medicine as We Saw It.* John E. Fogarty International Center for Advanced Study in the Health Sciences, 1974, 442 pp. U.S. Department of Health, Education and Welfare, Public Health Service National Institutes of Health, DHEW Publication No. (NIH) 75–684. This anthology is a collection of reports on China's medicine, written by American health professionals after their visits to the country in recent years. The book's five parts cover Chinese innovations in health, public health organization and practices, prevalent diseases in China, and biomedical research.

301　**Red Cross Societies,** *Report on the First Regional*

Red Cross Seminar for the Training of Auxiliary Health Workers in ther Rural Community. League of Red Cross Societies, Geneva, 1971, 8 pp. The problems discussed and conclusions reached by a seminar in Niamey, Niger, are set out in this document in the form of 'minutes'. They include brief descriptions of practical sessions demonstrating a simple method of filtering water in relation to prevention of cholera, and taking this demonstration into a selected village.

302 **Research Corporation,** *A Practical Guide to Combating Malnutrition in the Preschool Child.* Appleton Century-Crofts, New York, 1970, 74 pp. This report of a working conference on nutritional rehabilitation held at the National Institute of Nutrition, Bogota, Colombia, concludes that Nutritional Rehabilitation Centres should be part of a maternal and child welfare service but can operate in the absence of such a service. They are very suitable for staffing by auxiliaries and can be used as part of a training programme to extend a health centre's influence into the community.

303 **Rifkin, S. and Kaplinsky, R.,** *Health Strategy and Development Planning: Lessons from the People's Republic of China.* Journal of Development Studies (London), Vol. 9, No. 2, Jan. 1973, pp. 213–232. This is a very useful description and evaluation of the health services

in the People's Republic of China, which provide a comprehensive preventive programme for the greater part of the population. This has been achieved through mass campaigns for the eradication of communicable diseases and pests, the training and use of medical auxiliaries, and the incorporation of the traditional medical practitioners into the health system. Anyone interested in the planning of health services will find this book extremely useful.

304 **Rifkin, Susan B.,** *Who: How? (Helping People to Develop Community Health Programmes).* Christian Conference of Asia, Hong Kong, Jan. 1976, 28 pp. This unpublished document describes a programme to orientate all health workers, including doctors, to initiate community health programmes with the people. In five sessions it outlines integrated community based health programmes, understanding of group dynamics, dialogue with the community, programme planning and health education. Ideas for community diagnosis and teaching are appended with a short bibliography. Very useful for those involved in the training of health workers, and in any field of community development.

305 **Rogers, Everett,** *Communicación en las Campanas de Planificación Familiar* 1975, 700 pp. Translated from

Communication Strategies for Family Planning. Macmillan and Co., London. Intended for officials concerned with family planning programmes, this book is especially for those with responsibilities for providing large audiences with information, motivation, and education about contraception. It is also for researchers, teachers, and students with an interest in family planning communication.

306 **Ronaghy, H. A and Solter, S. L.,** *Auxiliary Health Worker in Iran,* The Lancet (London), Vol. 2, 25 August 1973, pp. 427–429. The health care needs of Iran's 55,000 villages are served by a system in which all medical graduates eligible for the army are drafted into rural health stations rather than military service. In theory, their work includes preventive medicine, health education, family planning, etc., but in practice it is limited to curative services. A 2-year pilot study was initiated to train, evaluate and discover the most effective role for 14 village health workers, and plans for a school for auxiliary health workers have received the approval of the Iranian Government.

307 **Ronaghy, Hossain A.** et al., *The Front Line Health Worker: Selection, Training and Performance.* American Journal of Public Health, (Washington), March 1976, Vol. 66, No. 3, pp. 273–277. This report describes the process of selection, training and deployment of auxiliary health workers and the levels of effort and productivity which may be expected of them after 6 months training. On the basis of their performance in 16 villages it was found that village health workers could effectively stimulate an awareness of the needs for environmental hygiene and sanitation improvements, and act as catalysts by taking specific action. Extremely useful for all programmes intending to use village health workers.

308 **Rosenfield, Allan G.,** *Auxiliaries and Family Planning.* Reprinted from The Lancet (London), Vol. 1, No. 7855, March 16, 1974, pp. 443–445. Available from The Population Council, New York. Auxiliaries can safely be used in family planning to provide services such as insertion of intrauterine contraceptive devices and prescription of oral contraceptives. In a pilot study in Thailand, auxiliary midwives prescribed the pill, using a medical checklist. This experiment was successful, and reached many additional acceptors, with no increase in side-effects or complications at follow-up one year later.

309 **Rowland, M. G. M., Cole, T. J. and Whitehead, R. G.,** *A Quantitative Study into the Role of Infection in Determining Nutritional Status in Gambian Village Children.* British Journal of Nutrition (London), Vol. 37, 1977, pp. 441–450. This study reports on the relationship

between the prevalence of nine different categories of disease and the growth of children measured in terms of weight and height for age. There was a significant negative relationship between gastroenteritis and both weight gain and height gain, and between malaria and weight gain only. Could be useful background material for training institutes.

310 **Rowley, John,** *We have survived another year.* People Magazine (London), Vol. 13, No. 2, 1976, pp. 17–24. This article describes the Danfa Project, an experimental rural health care project in 200 villages in the north of Accra in Ghana. Community participation is the key to the success of the experiment, and the project aims to investigate the best methods of providing health and family planning services, and to analyse the costs involved.

311 **Royal Society of Medicine and the Josiah Macy Foundation,** *The Greater Medical Profession.* Josiah Macy Foundation, New York, 1973, 258 pp. This book covers papers and discussions at a symposium which included representatives from medical education, medical practice, public health, dentistry, nursing, economics and sociology. The need for an increasing number and variety of health professionals to extend health care services throughout the world.

312 **Sadler, A. M., Sadler, B. L. and Bliss, A. A.,** *Physician's Assistant: Today and Tomorrow.* Yale University School of Medicine, New Haven Connecticut, U.S.A., 1972, 256 pp. The authors, a physician, a lawyer and a nurse, have combined to provide a unique view of issues which face the newest health care professional—the physician's assistant (PA). They acknowledge the value of the PA for improved health care, but point out the difficulties which may lie ahead, such as distribution, economics, education, delegation of tasks, and protection of the public. The emerging PA profession is urged to focus on the care of the patient. The authors do not profess to have simple answers to the issues they raise, but the book should produce dialogue and investigation into the improved care of patients.

313 **Said, Mohammed,** *Health Education and Preventive Medicine in the Community,* Hamdard National Foundation, Karachi, Pakistan. Paper presented at VI International Congress of Rural Medicine, Cambridge, U.K., 21–27 September 1975, 16 pp. The paper recommends that health education should be given to communities in order to improve community health. It stresses the need to use auxiliaries for community education, to use traditional medicine, and to change medical curricula in order to make them

more appropriate to the health needs of the country.

314 Sanders, R. K. M., *The Treatment of Tetanus with Intrathecal Antitetanus Serum.* Voluntary Health Association of India, New Delhi, 1977, 7 pp. This article describes the treatment of adult and neonatal tetanus patients with intrathecal antitetanus serum in rural Bihar, India. Principles in understanding and treating tetanus, and the estimation of potential mortality are described. Management of patients is covered in detail, with emphasis on nursing care and the administration of only 200 units of antitetanus serum by lumbar puncture. Such treatment has reduced the overall mortality among adult cases in the area to less than 5% over 2 years.

315 Saunders, Denys J., *Visual Communication Handbook: Teaching and Learning Using Simple Visual Materials.* United Society for Christian Literature, Lutterworth Press, London and Guildford, U.K., 1974, 127 pp. Also available from TALC (see entry 114). This well illustrated book is useful for trainers and communicators involved in fields of community development, agriculture, health and other social work. The book covers simple methods and techniques of production and utilization of visual materials. The principles, media and methods are appropriate for both rural and urban situations.

316 Schweser, Helen and Blaize, Agnes A., *The Development of a Health Education Department in a Less Developed Caribbean Country.* Project Hope, The People-to-People Health Foundation Inc., Washington, 1976, 70 pp. The authors emphasize the need to integrate health education into all fields of community development, and to coordinate all available methods of communication. The appendices outline outline in-service courses on health education for teachers and nurses. An extensive bibliography is included. Useful for trainers of auxiliaries on the planning of a community education strategy.

317 Silliman University Medical Center, *Workshop on Auxiliary Health Personnel.* Silliman University Medical Center, Dumaguete City, Philippines, 1975, 135 pp. The workshop aimed to define the role of health auxiliaries and to formulate programmes, policies, and recommendations related to them which may be incorporated into the national health plan. The report includes interesting papers such as 'Experiences and Observations on the Role of the Auxiliary Health Worker in Community Health', 'Justification for Utilization of Health Auxiliary and the Philippine Health System', and 'Some Issues Concerning the Use of Barangay Health Aides', as well as several information handouts, many group reports, and other useful data.

318 **Smith, R. A.,** *Towards Solving the Great Training Robbery.* The Pharos of Alpha Omega Alpha, U.S.A., Vol. 37, No. 2, 1974, pp. 47–52. A theoretical model is described that is designed to meet manpower needs in professions that are top-heavy with highly skilled professionals. This situation usually produces a lack of mid-level manpower, who potentially could increase the efficiency and productivity of these professions. Application of the theoretical model has been attempted in the MEDEX programme in the northern United States, and has proved so successful that broader application is suggested.

319 **Sox, Harold C. and Carol H. and Tompkins, R. K.,** *The Training of Physician's Assistants.* New England Journal of Medicine (Boston), April 1973, No. 288, pp. 818–824. This article suggests that a physician's assistant could evaluate 45% of patients correctly using a clinical flow chart system.

320 **Speight, A. N.,** *Cost-effectiveness and Drug Therapy.* Tropical Doctor (London), April 1975, pp. 89–92. The author states that Western prescribing habits are extravagant and wasteful especially in developing countries. Rural dispensaries lack essential drugs, while hospitals spend vast sums on them. He suggests methods for encouraging economic prescribing, proposing that journals require drug advertisements to contain prices of drugs advertised, and that the virtues of less expensive drugs should be widely disseminated to doctors by Ministries of Health.

321 **Spitzer, W. O.** et al., *The Burlington Randomized Trial of the Nurse Practitioner.* New England Journal of Medicine, Vol. 290, Jan. 31, 1974. The article shows that over 90% of patients in the trial were satisfied with medical auxiliary health care, and that the nurse-practitioner can cope unaided with approximately two thirds of all health problems.

322 **Standard, K. L.,** *Role of the Community Health Aide in the Commonwealth Caribbean, with Special Reference to Jamaica.* Paper presented at the International Medical and Research Foundation Symposium on the Community Health Worker, Warrenton, Virginia, U.S.A., 26–28 October, 1977, 17 pp. In 1967 the Department of Social and Preventive Medicine, University of West Indies, selected village residents for training as community health aides from two suburban low-income areas. The success of the programme encouraged the Ministry of Health and Environmental Control to train and employ 300 aides in 1972. By 1977 the number rose to 1,160 in the

Jamaican health services. The aides give health education, administer first aid, encourage family planning, check child immunization records, and are supervised by public health nurses.

323 **Stanley, Margaret,** *Two Experiences of an American Public Health Nurse in China, A Quarter of a Century Apart.* American Journal of Public Health (Washington), Vol. 63, No. 2, 1973, pp. 111–116. An American nurse tells of the dramatic changes in the Chinese health services between 1948 and 1972. She notes the absence of pests, the improvement in sanitation, the availability of family planning services, the emphasis on preventive health, the integration of Chinese and Western medicine, and the training of barefoot doctors. All these changes have contributed to the great improvement of the health of the Chinese people.

324 **Stolten, J. H. and Elman, A.,** *The Health Aide* Little, Brown and Co., Boston, U.S.A., 1972, 353 pp. Although prepared for the Health Aide in the United States as a training manual and reference source, this could be useful for other countries. It describes the basic skills required for the care of patients, the general care of infants, and includes material on task analysis, definitions, and procedures. Examples of work assignments which could help those charged with developing

training programmes are given. Well illustrated and produced.

325 **Sudan, Ministry of Health,** *Primary Health Care Programme: Southern Region Sudan 1977/78–1983/84.* Khartoum University Press, Khartoum, Sudan, Feb. 1976, 153 pp. This primary health care programme formulation document was produced in response to an urgent need to improve rural health care in the Southern Sudan. The study takes into account socioeconomic and political factors, and covers areas like health and development and participation, etc. Annexures include medical kits and standard equipment. Useful national planning document.

326 **Taylor, Carl E.,** *Health-Care Lessons from International Experience.* The New England Journal of Medicine (Boston), U.S.A., Vol. 290, No. 24, June 13, 1974, pp. 1376–1378. This short article defines the role of health auxiliaries and the advantages of using them to improve medical care. The author found that in India, auxiliaries in programmes produced multiple changes in health indices. For example, villages with auxiliaries had a 50% decline in child mortality compared with villages where government health centres were located, and doctors were in practice.

327 **Teik, Khoo Oon,** *Capabilities of Paramedical*

Personnel. Tropical Medicine and Public Health (Bangkok), Vol. 6, No. 2, June 1975, pp. 269–275. The article stresses the need to train paramedical personnel, auxiliaries and 'barefoot doctors' in order to respond to the needs of the neglected populations in the world. It reviews the performance and qualifications of these workers in various countries, and also includes a design for auxiliary training. Useful.

328   Thailand, Ministry of Public Health, *Guidelines for Development of the Village Health Volunteers Scheme.* Ministry of Public Health, Village Health Communicator and Village Health Volunteer Scheme, 1977–1981, Ministry of Public Health, Thailand, March 1977, 8 pp. Translated from Thai. The Thai Ministry of Health intends training a number of villagers who are interested in the health of their communities, and are willing to assist their neighbours as health communicators and health volunteers. The paper outlines the selection and role of these workers, and also the methods used in their training. Useful.

329   Théry, D., *Las Gaviotas Integrated Rural Development Centre.* Ecodevelopment News (Paris), No. 4, Feb. 1978, pp. 21–23. This report is an extract from a document which outlines the project in Las Gaviotas in Colombia. The project was established ten years ago to find a satisfactory means of providing incentives for settling the region without destroying its ecology. The article briefly describes the activities in the project of the Centre for Technological Development, which has produced many useful appropriate technology products such as a microturbine, a hand operated induction pump, a sail windmill, and a cassava grinder. The project hopes to set up a factory to manufacture these products.

330   Tichy, Monique K., *Behavioral Science Techniques: An Annotated Bibliography for Health Professionals.* Praeger Publishers, New York, 1975, 118 pp. With the emergence of interdisciplinary health care teams there is a need to prepare health workers to work effectively together during their training. This bibliography should prove most useful for trainers of any category of health worker. It includes sections on team development, techniques to improve group performance, and the evaluation of team training methods and their effectiveness. An extensive list of general references is included.

331   University of Dar es Salaam, Institute of Adult Education, *Mtu Ni Afya— Lifelong Education.* Institute of Adult Education, University of Dar es Salaam, Sept. 1972, 3 pp. This paper describes the aims of a health education scheme sponsored jointly by the Tanzanian Ministries of Health,

National Education, Regional Administration and Rural Development, and the Institute of Adult Education in 1972. Through the use of study groups and radio programmes, the scheme aimed to change people's attitudes towards disease and to bring about changes in personal and community habits which would lead to better health. Manuals about malaria and other infectious diseases were provided for village group leaders, and by May 1973 nearly two million adults were taking part in the studies.

332 **Upunda, G., Yudkin, J. and Brown, G.**, *Therapeutic Guidelines for Drug Usage in Tanzania.* 1977, 160 pp. This unpublished manual of therapeutic guidelines for use by doctors in Tanzania describes drug therapy for many different diseases, emphasizing the comparative costs of the different drugs available. It gives the correct dosages and administration of about 500 drugs, listed by generic rather than proprietary names. It also describes their side effects, and stresses the need for proper assessment of new drugs before they are prescribed.

333 **U.S.A. Department of Health, Education and Welfare,** *Health Auxiliary Training Instructor's Guide.* U.S. Department of Health, Education and Welfare, Division of Indian Health, Washington, 1966, 267 pp. The Division of Indian Health, in comprehensive health programmes for American Indians and Alaskan Natives, has found auxiliaries to be effective in meeting the health needs of the populations they serve. The manual covers all the important areas of public health such as epidemiology, basic home nursing, environmental health, etc. A suggested curriculum guide is included. Although written in 1966, this is a valuable manual for the planning and organization of a training programme.

334 **U.S.A., Department of Health, Education and Welfare,** *A Bibliography of Chinese Sources on Medicine and Public Health in the People's Republic of China 1960–1970.* U.S. Department of Health, Education and Welfare, John E. Fogarty International Center, Bethesda, U.S.A., 1973, 486 pp. This bibliography covers primarily those Chinese sources published between 1960 and 1970, translated from Chinese by the Joint Publications Research Service. One of the two sections covers articles from medical journals, magazines, and newspapers under two categories; clinical and health-related. The other section includes titles of books, monographs, and pamphlets on topics related to the bibliography.

335 **U.S.A., Department of Health, Education and Welfare,** *Topics of Study Interest in Chinese Medicine and Public*

Health: Report of a Planning Meeting. U.S. Department of Health, Education and Welfare, John E. Fogarty International Center, Bethesda, U.S.A., 1972, 85 pp. This summary of an informal planning meeting convened by the John E. Fogarty International Center contains reviews of ten topics in Chinese medicine and public health. These include discussions on the epidemiology of infections and parasitic diseases, population dynamics and family planning, and medical education, training and manpower.

336   **Van den Berghs & Jurgens Ltd.**, *Getting the Most Out of Food:* The twelfth in a series of studies on the modern approach to feeding and nutrition. Van den Berghs & Jurgens Ltd., Burgess Hill, West Sussex, U.K., 1977, 164 pp. This book contains some interesting prize winning essays which could be useful as background material for training institutes. Papers included are—'The Evaluation of a Nutrition Programme in Northern Ghana', 'Socioeconomic Differentials in Mortality', 'Can Severe Child Malnutrition be Prevented?', etc.

337   **van Etten, Gerardus Maria,** *Rural Health Development in Tanzania. A Case-study of Medical Sociology in a Developing Country. Proefschrift ter verkrijging van de graad van doctor in de Sociale Wetenschappen ann de Katholieke Universiteit to*

Nijmegen. Van Gorcum & Co., Assen, Netherlands, 1976, 182 pp. This is a sociological analysis of the constraints upon Tanzania's rural health development programme. Shortcomings of the existing health care system for rural areas, and the training and work situation of medical auxiliaries are seen as possible factors which are impeding rural health development. An entire chapter is dedicated to medical auxiliaries. Useful as good background material for trainers, and also for institutes for medical auxiliaries. A bibliography is included.

338   **Varma, S. K., Shrivastava, N. and Bole, S.V.,** *Artificial Aids for the Masses in the Developing Countries* in 'Disabled in Developing Countries', Commonwealth Foundation, London, 1977, pp. 36–38. This paper stresses the need for the development of inexpensive appropriate artificial aids for the disabled, which can be made by local artisans. It gives some examples such as a folding commode, cheap seats and tables, a modified lower leg prosthesis, a simple joint, and a cheap hand splint made from an aluminium clothes hanger.

339   **Viau, Alberto,** *Methodology for Training of Health Auxiliaries and its Impact on the Orientation for the Organization of the Health System.* Academy of Medical, Physical and Natural Sciences, Guatemala City, Guatemala,

1976, 40 pp. This paper analyses the delegation of tasks and the functions of health workers to make them appreciative of the health problems of the community. The application of systems analysis, operational research, occupational analysis, development of curricula, etc., have been utilized. This a highly technical paper which could be useful only for evaluators at national levels. An extensive bibliography is included.

340   Viau, A. and Croft Long, E., *The Training of Rural Health Workers in Guatemala and Their Relation to the Health System (Abstract).* Paper presented at the International Consultation on 'New types of basic health services worldwide and their implication for the education of other health care professionals', The Rockefeller Foundation Study and Conference Center, Bellagio, Italy, May 2–7, 1977, 8 pp. This paper reports on a pilot experiment to train rural health workers with the aim of integrating auxiliaries into the already existing services. The paper points out the advantages of training all categories of auxiliaries together. It covers the methods of training, supervision, and evaluation. Useful.

341   War on Want and Muller, Mike, *The Baby Killer.* War on Want, London, 1977, 23 pp. Also available from TALC (see entry 114). First published in 1974, this well informed and illustrated investigation into the deaths and damage caused by sales of powdered milks in the Third World has sparked off actions to ban the advertising of infant milks, as in Papua New Guinea and Guinea Bissau, and to promote breastfeeding campaigns. It has been translated (by other organizations) into German, French, Dutch, Danish, Spanish, Italian, and Swahili and this third edition includes an appendix containing additional discussion and references.

342   Watts, G., *People's Health in People's Hands.* World Medicine (London), Vol. 13, No. 8, 1978, pp. 19–23, 65, 67. The article reviews the Government of India's new health plan, which aims in the next three years to train one community health worker (CHW) for each of India's villages, which total over half a million. The plan includes the training of 100 community health workers in each of its 5,372 primary health centre (PHCs). The CHWs will combine preventive and curative roles, and will receive a simple medical kit and a manual for reference, with sections on traditional treatment. The plan also includes the training of traditional birth attendants and one male and one female multipurpose worker per 5,000 population. However, the problem of referral through health assistants, PHCs, and district hospitals must be solved if the system is to be efficient.

343 **Welty, T. K.,** *Navajo Community Health Representatives Programme.* International Medical and Research Foundation, Warrenton, Virginia, U.S.A., 1977, 8 pp. The Navajo community health representatives (CHRs) are trained to deal with the problems of the Indian people they serve. They are responsible for immunization, health education, local health schemes, home care plans, helping with emergency transport, and liaison between the Indians and the health service. The author feels that the CHR programme could be improved by providing vehicles with radios for the workers, and making schemes more adaptable to local conditions.

344 **Williams, Cicely D.,** *Foreword to Nutrition in the Community,* Edited by McLaren, D. S., John Wiley & Sons, London & New York, 1976, 23 pp. This interesting and thought-provoking foreword treats nutrition as a community problem. It analyses the difficulties experienced in other countries and the solutions often offered, such as mass feeding, supplementary programmes, and surveys. The need for future planning, which should include the training of auxiliaries and other appropriate health workers with a practical understanding of community nutrition, is emphasized. Useful as background material for trainers.

345 **Wingert, Willis A.** et al., *Effectiveness and Efficiency of Indigenous Health Aides in a Paediatric Outpatient Department.* American Journal of Public Health (Washington), Vol. 65, No. 8, August 1975, pp. 849–857. The article describes the use of indigenous health aides in California for the continued care of disadvantaged families, in order to provide effective services economically. It covers recruitment, a training programme, and an evaluation of their performance. Useful motivational and background material for trainers and also for training institutes.

346 **Wood, C. H.,** *Summary of the Current State of Community Health Workers in Kenya.* Presented at the International Medical and Research Foundation Symposium on the Community Health Worker, Warrenton, Virginia, U.S.A., 20–28 October, 1977, 3 pp. This paper describes the efforts being made both by the government and the voluntary agencies to improve the distribution of health services by outreach schemes, involving a variety of community health workers, which have recently been started in Kenya. Only one programme has been financially supported directly by the community. The author feels that often high salaries of health workers decrease the ability of local communities to fund their own programmes fully.

347 **World Health Organization,** *Approaches to Planning and Design of Health Care Facilities in Developing Areas.* (Volumes 1 and 2), Edited by Kleczkowski, B. M. and Pibouleau, R., World Health Organization, Geneva, 1976, 146 pp. This study has been undertaken by WHO to bridge the gap between existing knowledge and experience in design and architecture of hospitals and other medical care facilities in developing countries, and their practical utilization for health care planning and development. The study covers three main areas: legislative and administrative framework, planning and programming, and architecture and techniques. The study is well illustrated and many references are given.

348 **World Health Organization,** *Aspects of Medical Education in Developing Countries* by Ali, D. S. et al., WHO, Geneva, Public Health Papers No. 47, 1972, 116 pp. These selected papers deal with medical manpower and physician education in the Eastern Mediterranean region. They cover medical curricula, objectives of medical education in the developing countries, the integrated teaching of medical sciences, audiovisual media, etc. Particular mention is made of the problems of medical education in Iran.

349 **World Health Organization,** *Evaluation of Community Health Centres* by Roemer, M. I., WHO, Geneva, Public Health Papers No. 48, 1972, 42 pp. The various aspects and meanings of 'health centres' are described in this report. It reviews the literature on the evaluation of their activities, and recommends more research studies in the developing countries. Many references are included.

350 **World Health Organization,** *Final Report of the Regional Conference on Primary Health Care Manila, 21–24 November 1977.* Regional Office for the Western Pacific of the World Health Organization, Manila, Philippines, 1977, 68 pp. The report describes the conference's objectives and organization, and gives its recommendations on research and development, rural and urban development, community involvement, inter-sectoral approaches, manpower development, financing, and modification of the present health care delivery system. Annexes include guidelines for the preparation of country or area reports, summaries of actual reports, and discussions of critical issues in the implementation of primary health care.

351 **World Health Organization,** *Training of Medical Assistants and Similar Personnel.* WHO, Geneva, Technical Report series, No. 385, 1968, 26 pp. This report emphasizes the need for medical assistants in order to improve

health care in the community. It deals with training, objectives, curricula, teaching methods, etc. Examples illustrate training programmes in six countries—the Sudan, U.S.S.R., Algeria, Burma, Venezuela and the United States.

352 **World Health Organization,** *Training and Utilization of Village Health Workers.* WHO, Geneva, 1974, 324 pp. Available also in French and Spanish. The World Health Assembly, in 1972 and 1973, asked the World Health Organization to make an effort to assist in the improvement and extension of basic health services to rural populations in countries where this coverage is inadequate or non-existent. The village health worker—the first link in a health network—needs support and supervision, and a range of simple skills. Intended for adaptation to local conditions, and translation into local languages this document meets a well recognised need. Illustrated.

353 **World Neighbors,** *Audiovisual Communication Handbook.* Compiled and Edited by Dennis W. Pett, World Neighbors, Oklahoma City, Oklahoma, U.S.A., 1977, 125 pp. New edition from the original by Peace Corps, Washington. This manual is designed to assist educators to plan, produce and use instructional materials. Emphasis is given to materials which teachers can produce or obtain locally. The manual has five parts: planning instructional materials, use in the classroom and the community, presentation methods and materials, basic production techniques, and writing. There is an appendix with supplementary information and a limited index for reference.

354 **World Neighbors,** *Volunteer Health Promoters Can Form the Missing Link in Community Health.* World Neighbors in Action (Oklahoma City), Vol. 9, No. 1E, 1976, 8 pp. This article observes that volunteer health promoters actively participate in village development, and help their neighbours to solve community health problems. It describes a very successful project by the people in Purworejo-Klampok district in Central Java, Indonesia. It covers the appointment, training, and supervision of the volunteers, and also the work done by them in the community to improve the health of all. Well illustrated and useful.

355 **Wray, Joe D.,** *Health Maintaining Behaviour of Mothers in Traditional, Transitional and Modern Societies.* Paper prepared for session on Health Maintaining Behaviours, AAAS Meeting, New York City, January 1975, 44 pp. Available from the International Health Programs, Harvard School of Public Health, Boston, U.S.A. This interesting study shows the

excellent preparation for motherhood that a woman receives in a traditional society, as compared with that received by women living in urbanized areas. It discusses infant mortality, environmental factors, maternal diets, family size, etc. Good background for those interested in community health. An extensive list of references is given.

356   **Yemba, Konde Pambu,** *How a Rural Dispensary Becomes a Development Centre.* Contact (Geneva), No. 36, Dec. 1976, pp. 1–7. Reprinted in Appropriate Technology (London), Vol. 4, No. 1, May 1977, pp. 4–8. This article is a first-hand report of the experiences of a male nurse in charge of a dispensary in Sadi-Kinsanga in Zaire, who recognises the health needs and problems of the people he cares for. It describes how he encourages villagers to provide their own solutions. Good motivational material for auxiliaries. Describes the practical methods of community health work with village people.

357   **Yemen, Turba Rural Health Project,** *Turba Rural Health Project, Hugeriah District, Yeman Arab Republic: Programme Description.* Catholic Institute for International Relations, London, May 1976, 23 pp. This describes the development of the Turba rural health project within the socioeconomic situation of the Yemen. The booklet examines the project from its inception to its present state of development into a comprehensive community health programme, and the appendices include some valuable statistics.

Geographical Index

Africa, *see also specific country*
  1, 4, 6, 7, 22, 34, 35, 36, 38,
  43, 45, 51, 66, 71, 93, 119,
  145, 146, 148, 164, 167, 174,
  233, 243, 244, 247, 293
Alaska 2, 3, 11, 116, 228, 333
Algeria 351
Asia, *see also specific country* 7,
  167, 174, 233
Australia 149

Bangladesh 152, 153, 233
Botswana 183, 292
Burma 351

Cameroon 276
Canada 25, 26, 27, 28, 172, 173,
  257
Caribbean 106, 316
China 57, 61, 177, 181, 209,
  226, 272, 298, 300, 303, 323,
  334, 335
Colombia 30, 215, 329
Costa Rica 44, 138

Ethiopia 5, 148

Gambia 309
Ghana 161, 207, 310, 336
Guatemala 157, 266, 267, 289,
  339, 340

Honduras 170

India 48, 52, 53, 54, 70, 72, 78,
  121, 122, 123, 126, 169, 194,

229, 230, 231, 233, 235, 247,
  255, 263, 271, 277, 281, 294,
  314, 326, 342
Indonesia 55, 56, 94, 221, 233,
  279, 280, 283, 354
Iran 150, 151, 258, 306, 348
Ivory Coast 234

Jamaica 108, 159, 203, 236, 322
Java 221, 279, 280, 354

Kenya 246, 269, 270, 346
Korea, Republic of 182, 251

Latin America, *see also specific
  country* 42, 129, 167, 174,
  233, 247, 268
Lebanon 248
Lesotho 189, 259

Malagasy 190
Malawi 74, 75, 282
Malaysia 76, 77, 178
Mexico 41, 42, 95, 176, 220
Middle East, *see also specific
  country* 7, 150, 151

Nepal 14, 79, 80, 160, 180
Nigeria 34, 45, 287

Pakistan 313
Panama 199, 242
Papua New Guinea 12, 15, 81,
  83, 84, 85, 86, 92, 127, 136,
  137, 290

Peru 88, 135, 176, 215
Philippines 89, 104, 105, 317

Rhodesia 90

South Africa 217
South East Asia, *see under
specific country*
Sri Lanka 233, 238
Sudan 154, 156, 261, 325, 351

Tanzania 47, 112, 113, 130,
200, 209, 210, 223, 274, 331,
332, 337
Thailand 214, 296, 297, 308,
328

Uganda 29, 49

United Kingdom 31, 216
U.S.A. 8, 116, 158, 162, 212,
224, 256, 318, 324, 333, 343,
345, 351
U.S.S.R. 140, 351

Venezuela 120, 176, 241, 351

Western Samoa 24

Yemen 357

Zaire 32, 40, 58, 64, 96, 97, 98,
99, 100, 101, 117, 118, 141,
142, 165, 206, 237, 356
Zambia 68, 143, 144, 285

Subject Index

Administration 38, 51, 56, 65,
68, 88, 90, 113, 121, 148, 183,
191, 201, 224, 247, 259
Agent Sanitaire, *see under*
Auxiliary health worker
Aid post orderly, *see under*
Auxiliary health worker
Anaesthesia 119
Antenatal Care 2, 8, 28, 33, 35,
39, 41, 47, 72, 92, 122, 129,
136, 150, 156, 178, 200, 209,
234, 267
Anthropometric Measurement
9, 54, 66, 72, 96, 107, 159,
176, 188, 200, 229, 267, 309
Appropriate Technology 6, 7, 9,
17, 79, 124, 193, 204, 205,
222, 225, 232, 262, 269, 291,
329, 338
Audiovisual aid (or media) 42,
48, 72, 78, 114, 118, 121, 122,
123, 141, 160, 216, 225, 271,
315, 348, 353
Auxiliary Health Worker 1, 11,
12, 14, 15, 22, 25, 26, 30, 32,
33, 34, 39, 40, 41, 43, 44, 46,
47, 49, 50, 56, 60, 61, 65, 66,
70, 72, 73, 74, 75, 76, 79, 81,
83, 86, 87, 88, 90, 95, 106,
108, 110, 112, 113, 116, 119,
120, 122, 125, 126, 133, 136,
138, 139, 140, 148, 150, 151,
152, 153, 154, 157, 158, 163,
165, 169, 170, 171, 172, 173,
178, 180, 182, 183, 184, 189,
193, 197, 198, 199, 201, 209,

210, 212, 214, 215, 218, 220,
221, 223, 224, 226, 228, 232,
233, 235, 236, 237, 241, 242,
249, 251, 253, 255, 256, 275,
284, 288, 289, 292, 293, 294,
295, 296, 301, 306, 307, 312,
317, 319, 321, 322, 324, 326,
327, 331, 337, 339, 340, 351.
Auxiliary, Family Planning 42,
64, 152, 227, 298, 305, 308,
311
Auxiliary, Nurse 18, 22, 58, 70,
76, 80, 83, 88, 135, 147, 169,
173, 178 217, 234, 267, 321

Barefoot Doctor, *see under*
Community health worker
Basic health worker, *see under*
Auxiliary health worker
Birth control, *see under Family*
Planning
Breastfeeding 72, 122, 212, 273,
341, 355
Building 31, 124, 232, 347

Child Health 9, 12, 13, 15, 20,
23, 28, 29, 34, 35, 36, 37, 41,
48, 49, 53, 54, 55, 59, 60, 63,
65, 68, 70, 72, 80, 81, 86, 99,
105, 107, 121, 122, 129, 132,
137, 139, 159, 163, 170, 176,
178, 192, 195, 209, 217, 222,
229, 231, 236, 254, 266, 267,
270, 273, 278, 281, 282, 302,
309, 324, 341
Communicable diseases 14, 15,

18, 43, 53, 74, 80, 82, 97, 102,
109, 117, 118, 139, 163, 185,
195, 211, 245, 299, 309, 311,
314
Communications 25, 78, 101,
114, 121, 146, 172, 194, 196,
204, 224, 225, 228, 246, 252,
262, 271, 305, 315, 353
Community development 48,
115, 139, 152, 153, 157, 179,
202, 204, 232, 238, 241, 248,
250, 279, 294, 311, 316, 325,
329, 350, 357
Community diagnosis 9, 40, 48,
51, 66, 149, 155, 179, 219,
263, 270, 283, 299
Community health, *see also*
Primary health care 1, 3, 22,
26, 43, 44, 48, 52, 56, 66, 73,
77, 104, 105, 106, 108, 113,
116, 121, 123, 126, 139, 146,
150, 151, 152, 153, 154, 155,
157, 160, 161, 168, 170, 174,
176, 179, 180, 182, 184, 185,
186, 195, 202, 206, 213, 215,
219, 220, 229, 233, 238, 251,
257, 258, 259, 263, 273, 274,
279, 280, 281, 283, 285, 294,
297, 304, 307, 310, 311, 313,
317, 322, 328, 343, 345, 346,
352, 354, 356, 357
Community health aide, *see*
under Community health
worker
Community health worker 3,
14, 15, 25, 26, 27, 30, 36, 44,
48, 52, 53, 56, 60, 61, 63, 66,
72, 88, 105, 108, 116, 122,
126, 135, 137, 138, 150, 151,
152, 153, 157, 159, 170, 172,
173, 180, 181, 182, 189, 206,
215, 220, 221, 226, 233, 242,
251, 253, 255, 258, 259, 260,
261, 270, 274, 279, 280, 281,
287, 292, 297, 307, 317, 322,
326, 328, 342, 343, 345, 346,
352, 354, 356

Community nurse, *see under*
Nurse and Auxiliary Nurse
Community Participation 24,
48, 94, 98, 106, 117, 129, 146,
152, 153, 157, 160, 167, 169,
170, 172, 192, 199, 206, 209,
220, 221, 230, 233, 234, 242,
246, 251, 258, 279, 280, 281,
304, 310, 331, 346, 356
Construction, *see under Building*
Cost-benefit analysis, *see under*
Health economics
Culture, *see under*
Socio-economic
Curriculum 2, 4, 11, 18, 30, 48,
50, 76, 94, 112, 113, 120, 126,
140, 148, 165, 183, 201, 217,
222, 234, 261, 286, 296, 316,
327, 331, 348, 351

Dental Health 24, 46, 128, 223,
275, 288, 296
Diagnosis 9, 20, 38, 40, 61, 66,
75, 79, 81, 107, 109, 122, 130,
133, 147, 163, 166, 200, 211,
255, 319
Diarrhoea 13, 29, 60, 72, 81,
122, 245, 266, 273, 309
Disease control 4, 21, 26, 56, 82,
117, 155, 163, 164, 170, 180,
190, 195, 206, 207, 238, 242,
245, 261, 273, 311, 314
Dispensary 45, 58, 163, 320,
332, 356
Doctor 38, 51, 106, 132, 147,
154, 166, 197, 201, 254, 289
Drugs 14, 31, 32, 44, 53, 60, 70,
85, 90, 127, 133, 143, 147,
190, 193, 320, 332

Emergency medical care 10, 16,
17, 111, 112, 128, 132, 248,
299
Environmental health 10, 21,
26, 44, 48, 52, 74, 77, 86, 102,
105, 108, 117, 120, 121, 124,
129, 135, 139, 150, 170, 180,

190, 206, 215, 219, 232, 238,
242, 279, 280
Equipment 7, 31, 67, 79, 85, 88,
93, 185, 192, 232, 262, 267,
291, 325, 329, 338, 347
Evaluation 78, 125, 126, 134,
149, 150, 151, 171, 175, 191,
199, 217, 247, 250, 263, 289,
303, 307, 330, 340, 345, 349
Eye disease 75, 103, 110

Family planning 33, 41, 42, 61,
64, 79, 80, 84, 89, 90, 91, 129,
152, 153, 174, 191, 194, 227,
246, 247, 268, 298, 305, 308
First aid, see also Emergency
medical care 16, 17, 30, 111
Food technology 23, 59, 66, 68,
71, 115, 124, 152, 153, 186,
205, 230, 232, 269

Government programme 11, 25,
26, 52, 56, 57, 76, 77, 79, 80,
140, 150, 151, 154, 160, 170,
172, 177, 178, 183, 191, 194,
207, 210, 214, 221, 233, 242,
251, 252, 256, 258, 259, 272,
274, 276, 283, 290, 296, 300,
303, 306, 317, 322, 323, 325,
328, 331, 334, 335, 337, 342,
350, 351

Handbook, see under Training
and Reference manuals;
teaching aid
Health Assistant, see under
Auxiliary health worker
Health centre 31, 33, 45, 55, 56,
65, 69, 80, 88, 93, 112, 113,
120, 135, 138, 143, 152, 153,
158, 162, 189, 235, 274, 342,
349
Health economics 31, 57, 151,
183, 189, 222, 278, 280, 289,
291, 310, 312, 320, 346, 349,
350
Health education 5, 12, 22, 29,

30, 56, 58, 63, 68, 72, 91, 94,
96, 97, 98, 99, 100, 101, 106,
113, 114, 118, 121, 122, 123,
129, 130, 131, 141, 142, 146,
159, 160, 169, 170, 182, 194,
198, 199, 203, 206, 215, 216,
231, 236, 242, 246, 247, 250,
255, 257, 270, 273, 283, 287,
297, 304, 305, 311, 313, 315,
316, 322, 328, 331, 343, 348,
351
Health insurance 152, 153, 221,
279, 280
Health manpower 11, 57, 69,
76, 134, 145, 154, 167, 171,
173, 176, 187, 197, 198, 200,
208, 210, 214, 222, 232, 233,
237, 241, 243, 247, 249, 263,
264, 276, 284, 288, 293, 311,
318, 348, 350
Health team 24, 45, 48, 65, 104,
152, 153, 184, 197, 223, 233,
243, 256, 276, 288, 330
Hospital 46, 158, 189, 199, 206,
208, 232, 234, 279
Hygiene 21, 27, 61, 63, 129,
131, 142, 156, 178, 180, 189,
266

Immunization 44, 54, 60, 63,
105, 215, 246, 273, 278, 322,
343
Infant feeding 20, 23, 28, 35,
36, 49, 59, 66, 72, 74, 122,
137, 156, 169, 176, 229, 230,
239, 240, 273, 341, 344
Infectious diseases, see under
Communicable diseases;
disease control; skin diseases
International organization 151,
169, 179, 180, 254, 262

Job description 4, 11, 76, 145,
154, 173, 215, 237, 249, 259,
274, 287, 289, 295, 296, 307,
317, 322, 324, 327, 328, 339

88

Laboratory 31, 56, 67, 93, 127, 296

Leprosy 4, 5, 6, 7, 19, 63, 86, 87, 103, 130, 147, 148, 164, 166, 185, 245, 255

Malnutrition 9, 20, 49, 59, 68, 69, 71, 72, 81, 90, 102, 103, 107, 122, 144, 159, 169, 203, 229, 230, 244, 250, 266, 282, 302, 336, 341

Maternal child health, *see also Antenatal care; child health; infant feeding; obstetrics* 12, 15, 27, 28, 30, 33, 37, 41, 44, 47, 48, 52, 68, 69, 72, 77, 79, 80, 84, 86, 94, 96, 105, 108, 121, 122, 137, 139, 146, 150, 174, 178, 180, 195, 200, 203, 209, 219, 229, 234, 239, 240, 246, 250, 251, 254, 258, 261, 267, 273, 278, 279, 280, 281, 292, 302, 322, 355

Medex, *see under Auxiliary health worker*

Medical assistant, *see under Auxiliary health worker*

Medical records 28, 38, 54, 68, 88, 105, 112, 200, 219, 250, 273, 319

Mental health 52, 162, 185, 236

Midwife 2, 8, 33, 35, 37, 39, 41, 45, 48, 77, 84, 122, 123, 136, 156, 178, 293, 297, 308

Mobile services 24, 158, 189, 213, 234, 260, 273

Nurse 2, 8, 15, 19, 32, 34, 58, 76, 81, 83, 85, 86, 90, 91, 106, 173, 212, 217, 227, 283, 286, 321, 356

Nurse midwife 2, 8, 33, 37, 39, 70, 76, 80, 84, 136, 178, 212

Nutrition 9, 12, 20, 23, 48, 49, 56, 59, 60, 63, 66, 68, 69, 71, 72, 74, 75, 78, 80, 86, 96, 105, 108, 115, 122, 137, 144, 159, 169, 174, 176, 180, 186, 188, 189, 195, 203, 205, 215, 219, 229, 230, 231, 234, 239, 240, 247, 250, 266, 267, 270, 272, 273, 278, 287, 302, 309, 336, 341, 344

Obstetrics 8, 33, 35, 39, 41, 47, 75, 77, 80, 84, 86, 90, 92, 112, 129, 136, 156, 200, 267, 286

Parasitic diseases 102, 117, 118, 190, 245, 266, 309

Pest control 21, 26

Physician, *see under Doctor*

Planning 51, 54, 57, 65, 68, 82, 115, 126, 154, 155, 183, 185, 186, 187, 189, 195, 201, 207, 209, 212, 218, 229, 232, 247, 250, 259, 273, 290, 291, 304, 317, 347

Preventive health 1, 3, 12, 30, 45, 48, 58, 73, 95, 99, 129, 133, 142, 146, 152, 153, 170, 177, 181, 190, 195, 210, 215, 258, 273, 274, 279, 303, 313, 323, 333

Primary health care, *see also Community health* 11, 52, 70, 139, 150, 151, 152, 153, 154, 155, 158, 162, 167, 174, 176, 181, 182, 183, 184, 189, 198, 199, 200, 206, 207, 209, 210, 233, 237, 238, 242, 245, 252, 258, 261, 264, 284, 289, 290, 291, 294, 300, 303, 306, 312, 317, 323, 325, 328, 334, 335, 339, 342, 347, 350, 352

Rehabilitation 4, 6, 18, 68, 164, 185, 236, 250, 260, 302, 338

Research 149, 151, 158, 161, 176, 181, 187, 188, 203, 208, 266, 267, 289, 300, 309, 321, 339, 355

Rural health post, *see under Health centre*

Rural health promoter, *see under Auxiliary health worker*

Sanitation 10, 21, 26, 74, 102, 117, 120, 124, 135, 139, 180, 206, 215, 219, 232, 270, 279, 280
School health 5, 36, 74, 96, 97, 98, 100, 101, 144, 273
Screening, *see under Diagnosis*
Skin diseases 43, 75, 103
Socio-economic 48, 57, 152, 153, 157, 176, 177, 186, 187, 188, 191, 195, 200, 203, 218, 232, 239, 267, 273, 278, 311, 325, 336, 337, 355, 357
Supervision 4, 48, 148, 165, 171, 180, 201, 340, 354
Surgery 43, 119, 121, 211
Survey 9, 128, 149, 187, 256, 263, 284

Teaching aid 5, 26, 42, 48, 63, 72, 78, 114, 116, 118, 121, 122, 141, 160, 175, 216, 255, 271, 314, 348, 353
Therapy 13, 14, 29, 49, 54, 60, 62, 65, 87, 109, 127, 143, 147, 166, 190, 211, 332
Traditional birth attendant 2, 39, 123, 129, 156, 178, 342
Traditional medicine 52, 60, 123, 129, 161, 176, 203, 218, 238, 277, 303, 313, 342
Traditional practitioner 129, 161, 203, 218, 220, 238, 277, 303, 342
Training, *see also Training, auxiliary health worker; Training, community health worker* 2, 4, 5, 51, 54, 77, 89, 91, 104, 134, 145, 160, 174, 175, 196, 204, 217, 231, 234, 243, 264, 276, 286, 316, 330
Training, auxiliary health worker 3, 11, 12, 30, 40, 48, 50, 66, 70, 76, 86, 95, 108, 112, 113, 116, 118, 120, 125, 126, 131, 139, 140, 150, 158, 165, 170, 171, 172, 173, 178, 183, 201, 224, 237, 292, 296, 301, 307, 317, 324, 327, 333, 337, 339, 340, 351
Training, community health worker 3, 40, 48, 66, 108, 116, 123, 126, 129, 150, 156, 170, 172, 173, 258, 281, 287, 292, 307, 317, 328, 345, 352, 354
Training and reference manuals, *see also training and reference manuals, auxiliary health worker; training and reference manuals, community health worker* 2, 4, 6, 7, 16, 17, 18, 51, 58, 84, 85, 89, 91, 92, 93, 104, 111, 115, 130, 132, 286
Training and reference manuals, auxiliary health worker 11, 12, 14, 15, 22, 23, 25, 26, 30, 32, 33, 39, 41, 43, 44, 55, 56, 61, 62, 70, 75, 79, 80, 81, 86, 87, 88, 90, 106, 108, 112, 113, 116, 120, 133, 136, 138, 139, 172, 324
Training and reference manuals, community health worker 3, 14, 15, 25, 26, 27, 30, 44, 52, 53, 56, 61, 63, 88, 105, 108, 116, 129, 135, 137, 138, 172
Tuberculosis 82, 109, 211, 245

Underfives' clinic 31, 49, 54, 55, 195, 219, 273, 278, 281, 282, 292

Village health worker, *see under community health worker*
Voluntary organization 152, 157, 160, 169, 180, 183, 206, 220, 221, 233, 238, 262, 263, 285, 292
Water supply 10, 26, 124, 190, 232, 269, 301

Useful Addresses

AFGHANISTAN

Public Health Institute, Kabul, Afghanistan.

ARGENTINA

Department of Social Welfare, Buenos Aires, Argentina.

AUSTRALIA

Aboriginal Medical Service, Alice Springs, NT 5750, Australia.

Community Health Services, Department of Public Health, P.O. Box 265, West Perth, Western Australia 6005.

UNICEF—Australia & New Zealand Region, P.O. Box 4045, G.P.O. Sydney, Australia.

University of New South Wales, P.O. Box 1, Kensington, New South Wales, Australia 2033.

University of Sydney, School of Public Health & Tropical Medicine, New South Wales, Australia 2006.

University of Western Australia, Department of Microbiology, Perth Medical Centre, Shenton Park, Western Australia 6008.

BANGLADESH

Christian Commission for Development in Bangladesh (CCDB), Road 18, Dhanmandi RA, Dacca, Bangladesh.

Concern Bangladesh, P.O. Box 650, House 283, Road 26, Dhanmandi, Dacca 5, Bangladesh.

Gonashasthaya Kendra, P.O. Nayarhat, District Dacca, Bangladesh.

Rural Health Project, Bassurhal, P.S. Companiganj, District Noakhali, Bangladesh.

Rural Health Research Centre, P.O. Box 367, House 615, Road 18, Dacca, Bangladesh.

BELGIUM

Ecole de Santé Publique, Université Catholique de Louvain, 4 Avenue Chapelle aux Champs, 1200 Brussels, Belgium.

Institut de Médecine Tropicale Prince Leopold, Nationalestraat 155, 2000 Antwerp, Belgium.

BOLIVIA

Madres de Caridad, Casilla 2329, La Paz, Bolivia.

Ministerio de Prevision Social y Salud Publica, Division Nacional de Enfermeria, La Paz, Bolivia.

BOTSWANA

International Planned Parenthood Federation, Family Welfare Office, Department of Medical Services, Private Bag No. 38, Gaberone, Botswana.

BRAZIL

Associacao Sulina de Credito e Assistencia Rural (ASCAR), Rua Siquera Campos 1184, Lo Andar, P.O. Box 2727, Porto Algre, RS, Brazil.

Escola Paulista de Medicine, Departmento de Medicina Preventiva, (Vila Clementina), Rua Botucatu 720, Caize Postal 7144, Sao Paulo, Brazil.

Fundacao W.K. Kellogg Para a America Latina, Rua Mexico, 41 Sala 704, Rio de Janeiro, GB, Brazil.

Ministerio de Saude, Fundacao Servicios de Saude Publica, Avenue Rio Branco 251, Rio de Janeiro, Brazil.

CAMEROON, United Republic of

African Health Training Institutions Project, University Centre for Health Science, Yaounde, United Republic of Cameroon.

CANADA

Canadian International Development Agency (CIDA), 122 Bank Street, Ottawa, Canada KIA OG4

Canadian Universities Service Overseas (CUSO), 151 Slater Street, Ottawa, Ontario, K1P 5H5, Canada.

92

Department of Education Planning, 6th Floor, 252 Bloor Street West, Toronto, Ontario, Canada M5S 1V6.

Department of National Health & Welfare, 255 Argyle Avenue, Ottawa, Ontario, Canada M5S 1V6.

Department of National Health & Welfare, Publications Department, Brooke-Claxton Building, Ottawa K1A 0K9, Canada.

Department of National Health & Welfare, Saskatchewan Region. Medical Services, 500 Derrick Building, 2431 11th Avenue, Regina, Saskatchewan S4P 0K4, Canada.

International Development Research Centre, P.O. Box 8500, Ottawa, K1G 3H9, Canada.

CHILE

Servico Nacional de Salud, Sección de Acción Communitaria y Salud Rural, Santiago, Chile.

UNICEF—Regional Office of the Americas, Avenida Isidora Goyenechea 3322, Cassilla 13970, Santiago, Chile.

COLOMBIA

Estudio Experimental de Servicios de Salud, Oficina de Administración de Recursos Humanos, Bogota, Colombia.

International Centre for Medical Research & Training, Aptdo Aeri 5390, Cali, Colombia.

Ministerio de Salud Publica, Division de Atención Medica, Bogota D.E., Colombia.

Pan American Federation of Associations of Medical Schools, Carrera 7 No. 29–34, Bogota, D.E., Colombia.

Programa de Investigaciónes en Planeación de Salud, Apartado Aereo 4074, Cali, Colombia.

CONGO

World Health Organization Regional Office for Africa, P.O. Box 6, Brazzaville, Congo.

COSTA RICA

Ministry of Health Education, San Jose, Costa Rica.

CYPRUS

Near East Ecumenical Committee for Palentine Refugees, P.O. Box 4047, Nicosia, Cyprus.

DAHOMEY

Maternal and Child Health Project, University of California Extension, B.P. 119, Cotonou, Dahomey.

DENMARK

World Health Organization Regional Office for Europe, 8, Scherfigsvej, 2100 Copenhagen Ø, Denmark.

EGYPT

World Health Organization Regional Office for the Eastern Mediterranean, P.O. Box 1517, Alexandria, Egypt.

EIRE

The Medical Missionaries of Mary, International Missionary Training Hospital, Drogheda, Co. Louth, Eire.

ETHIOPIA

All Africa Leprosy & Rehabilitation Training Centre (ALERT), P.O. Box 165, Addis Ababa, Ethiopia.

Ministry of Public Health, Medical Services Division, P.O. Box 1234, Addis Ababa, Ethiopia.

FIJI

Fiji School of Medicine, Suva, Fiji.

South Pacific Health Service Publications, Nutrition Section, Suva, Fiji.

FRANCE

Centre International de L'Enfance, Chateau de Longchamp, Bois de Boulogne, 75016 Paris, France.

94

Organisation for Economic Cooperation & Development (OECD), Development Centre, 94 rue Chardon-Lagache, 75016 Paris, France.

GHANA

Ghana Medical School, Department of Preventive Medicine, P.O. Box 4236, Accra, Ghana.

Ministry of Health, Accra, Ghana.

University of Ghana, Department of Sociology, Legon, Accra, Ghana.

GUATEMALA

Clinica Behrhorst, Apartado 15, Chimaltenango, Guatemala, C.A.

Division of Applied Nutrition, INCAP, Carretera Roosevelt Zona 11, Apartado Postal 1188, Guatemala, C.A.

Mission del Quiche, El Convento, Chichicastenango, Guatemala, C.A.

HONDURAS

Cuerpo de Paz in Honduras, Apto Post C-51, Teguci Galpa, Honduras.

El Programa de Promotoras de Salud, Olancho, Honduras, C.A.

HONG KONG

Centre of Asian Studies, University of Hong Kong, Pokfulam Road, Hong Kong.

Christian Conference of Asia, c/o Hong Kong Christian Council, 57 Peking Road 4/F, Kowloon, Hong Kong.

Department of Preventive and Social Medicine, University of Hong Kong, Li Shu Fan Building, Sassoon Road, Hong Kong.

INDIA

All India Institute of Medical Sciences, Ansari Nagar, New Delhi 110 016, India.

Central Health Education Bureau, Kotla Road, New Delhi 110 016, India.

Christian Medical Association of India, Christian Council Lodge, Nagpur 440 001, Madya Pradesh, India.

Community Health Project, Victoria Hospital, Dichpalli P.O., Nizamabad District, Andhra Pradesh, India.

Comprehensive Rural Health Project, Marathi Church Mission, Jamkhed, Maharashtra, India.

Department of Paediatrics, University of Chandigarh, Punjab, India.

Director-General of Health Services, Nirman Bhavan, New Delhi 110 001, India.

Emmanuel Hospitals Association, 808/92 Nehru Place, New Delhi 110 024, India.

Gandhigram Institute of Rural Health & Family Planning, P.O. Ambathurai R.S., District Madurai, Tamil Nadu 624 309, India.

Indian Council for Child Welfare, 4 Dean Dyal Upadhyaya Marg, New Delhi 110 001, India.

Indian Council of Medical Research, Ansari Nagar, New Delhi 110 016, India.

Indo-Dutch Project for Child Welfare, 63–885 Somaljiguda, Hyderabad, Andhra Pradesh 500 004, India.

Jawaharlal Institute of Postgraduate Medical Education and Research, Pondicherry, Tamil Nadu 665 006, India.

The Leprosy Mission, c/o Philadelphia Leprosy Hospital, Salur, Andhra Pradesh 532 591, India.

Medico Friends Circle, 21 Nirman Society, Vadodara, Gujarat 390 005, India.

Ministry of Health & Family Welfare, Nirman Bhavan, New Delhi 110 001, India.

National Environmental Engineering Research Institute, Nehru Marg, Nagpur, Madya Pradesh 440 020, India.

National Institute of Health and Family Welfare, L 17 Green Park, New Delhi 110 016, India.

National Institute of Nutrition, Hyderabad, Andhra Pradesh 500 007, India.

Rural Health Research Centre (R.H.R.C.), Narangwal, District Ludhiana, Punjab, India.

Tuberculosis Association of India, 3 Red Cross Road, New Delhi 110 001, India.

UNICEF—South Central Asia Regional Office, 11 Jor Bagh, New Delhi 110 001, India.

Voluntary Health Association India, C 14 Community Centre, Safdarjung Development Area, New Delhi 110 016, India.

World Health Organization Regional Office for South-East Asia,

World Health House, Indraprastha Estate, Ring Road, New Delhi 110 001, India.

INDONESIA

Bureau of Education & Training, Ministry of Health, Parapattan 10, Jakarta, Indonesia.

Council of Churches in Indonesia, Department of Service & Development, Jalan Dempo 3, Jakarta Pusat, Indonesia.

Directorate General of Community Health, Ministry of Health, Parapattan 10, Jakarta, Indonesia.

Division on Health & Responsible Parenthood, Council of Churches in Indonesia, Jalan Dempo 3, Jakarta Pusat, Indonesia.

Lembaga Kesehatan Nasional, Jl. Perceraken Negara No.1, Jakarta, Indonesia.

Ministry of Education & Culture, Consortium of Medical Sciences, 6 Selamba, Jakarta, Indonesia.

Panti Walujo Hospital, Solo, Central Java, Indonesia.

IRAN

Department of Community Medicine, Pahlavi University School of Medicine, Shiraz, Iran.

Health Corps Organization, Ministry of Health, 258 Shah Street, Teheran, Iran.

Imperial Organization for Social Services, Teheran, Iran.

Institute of Public Health Research, P.O. Box 1310, Teheran, Iran.

Iran-WHO International Epidemiological Research Centre, Institute of Public Health Research, P.O. Box 1555, Teheran, Iran.

ISRAEL

University of Negev, P.O. Box 2053, Beer-Sheva, Israel.

ITALY

Food & Agriculture Organization (FAO), Publications Division, Via delle Terme di Caracalla, 00100 Rome, Italy.

IVORY COAST

UNICEF—Regional Office for West Africa, P.O. Box 4443, Abidjan Plateau, Ivory Coast.

JAMAICA

The Caribbean Institute on Mental Retardation & Development Disabilities, 2D Suthermere Road, Kingston, Jamaica.

University of West Indies, Department of Social & Preventive Medicine, Mona Kingston, 7 Jamaica.

JAPAN

UNICEF—Regional Office, Shin Ohtemachi, 2 Chome, Tokyo 100, Japan.

JORDAN

University of Amman, School of Nursing, Amman, Jordan.

KENYA

African Medical & Research Foundation, P.O. Box 30125, Nairobi, Kenya.

East African Leprosy Association, P.O. Box 30644, Nairobi, Kenya.

East Africa Literature Bureau, P.O. Box 3002, Nairobi, Kenya.

Food & Agriculture Organization, Box 30470, Nairobi, Kenya.

Medical Training Centre, P.O. Box 30195, Nairobi, Kenya.

Medical Training School, P.O. Box 10042, Nakuru, Kenya.

UNICEF—Regional Office for East Africa, P.O. Box 44145, Nairobi, Kenya.

University of Nairobi, Department of Paediatrics, Faculty of Medicine, P.O. Box 30588, Nairobi, Kenya.

KOREA, Republic of

School of Public Health, Seoul National University, Yon Keun Dong 28, Seoul, Republic of Korea.

LEBANON

UNICEF—Regional Office for Eastern Mediterranean, P.O. Box 5902, Beirut, Lebanon.

LESOTHO

St James Mission Hospital, Mants'onyane, Lesotho.

98

MALAWI

Ministry of Extension & Training, Ministry of Agriculture & Natural Resources, Lilongwe, Malawi.

Extension Aids Officer, Box 250, Zomba, Malawi.

Ministry of Health, P.O. Box 95, Blantyre, Malawi.

Private Hospital Association of Malawi, P.O. Box 948, Blantyre, Malawi.

MALAYSIA

Hospital Assistant Training School, Sarawak General Hospital, Kuching, Sarawak, Malaysia.

Instit Penyelidikan Perubatan, International Centre for Medical Research, University of California, Kuala Lumpur, Malaysia.

Ministry of Health, Jalan Young, Kuala Lumpur, Malaysia.

University of Malaya, Department of Social & Preventive Medicine, Kuala Lumpur, Malaysia.

MAURITIUS

School of Agriculture, University of Mauritius, Redult, Mauritius.

MEXICO

Academia Hispano Americana, Insurgentes 21, San Miguel de Allende, G.T.O., Mexico.

Associación Mexicana Albert Schweitzer, Bahia de Ballenas No. 88-2, Mexico 17, D.F.

Community Medicine Program, Pino 23, Mexico 21, D.F.

Centre de Estudios Generales, A.C., Aptdo 732, Chihuahua, Chih, Mexico.

Dirección General de Servicios Coordinados de Salud Publica, 436 Edificio 10, Entrada 3, Depto 707, Unidad Nonoalco, Tlatelolco, Mexico, D.F.

Editorial Pax-Mexico, Libreria Carlos Cesarman, S.A., Apartado Postal 45-009, Mexico, D.F.

Mexican Society of Public Health, Cancum, Mexico.

National Universidad Autonomo de Mexico, Facultad de Medicine, Mexico, D.F.

Nueva Editorial Interamericana, S.A. de C.V. Cedro, 512 Mexico 4, D.F., Mexico.

Servicios Educativos Populares A.C., Aptdo Postal 57, Cd Nezahualcoyotl, Edo. De Mexico, Mexico.

Servicio Nacional Penitenceria, Mexico, D.F.

MOZAMBIQUE

Ministerio de Saude, B.P. 264, Maputo, Mozambique.

NEPAL

Department of Health Services, Ministry of Health, Kathmandu, Nepal.

Ministry of Health, Training Cell, Community Health & Integration of Health Services Division, Department of Health Services, Kathmandu, Nepal.

Shanta Bhawan Hospital, Box 252, Kathmandu, Nepal.

NETHERLANDS

Academisch Ziekenhuis-Leiden, Rijnsburgerweg 10, Postrekening 425162, Leiden, The Netherlands.

Algemeen Provinciaal, Stads-En Academisch Zeikenhuis, Oogheelkundige Kliniek, Oostersingel 59, Groningen, The Netherlands.

Netherlands Reformed Church Missionary Council, POB 12, Oegstgeest, Leidsestraatweg 11, The Netherlands.

Royal Tropical Institute, Department of Tropical Hygiene, 63 Mauritskade, Amsterdam-Oost, The Netherlands.

NICARAGUA

Medico, Managua, Nicaragua.

NIGER

Ministry of Health, Government of Niger, Niamey, Niger.

NIGERIA

Christian Council of Nigeria, Ikot Ibritam, PMB 38, Abak, South Eastern States, Nigeria.

Medical Auxiliaries Training School, Sudan Interior Mission, Jos, Nigeria.

Ministry of Health, Kaduna, Northern Nigeria, Nigeria.

100

Ministry of Health, Public Health Department, Ibadan, Nigeria.

St. Luke's Hospital, Annua-Uyo, South Eastern State, Nigeria.

UNICEF—Regional Office for Nigeria & Ghana, P.O. Box 1282, Lagos, Nigeria.

University of Lagos, Institute of Child Health, Health Centre Building, Randle Avenue, Surulere, P.M.B. 1001, Lagos, Nigeria.

NORWAY

Freedom from Hunger Campaign-Action for Development, Pilestredet 57, Box 8139 Oslo-Dept, Oslo 1, Norway.

Nutrition Institute, University of Oslo, Blindern, Oslo 3, Norway.

PAKISTAN

Hamdard National Foundation, Nazimabad, Karachi 18, Pakistan.

PANAMA

Hospital de Changuinola, Bocas del Toro, Panama.

Ministerio de Salud, Departmento de Impression y Publicaciónes, Panama.

PAPUA NEW GUINEA

Department of Public Health, P.O. Box 2084, Konedobu, Papua New Guinea.

Nursing Education Division, Department of Public Health, P.O. Box 2084, Konedobu, Papua New Guinea.

Papua New Guinea Paramedical College, P.O. Box 1034, Boroko, Papua New Guinea.

Paramedical College, Department of Public Health, P.O. Box 2033, Yomba, Madang, Papua New Guinea.

Port Moresby General Hospital, Boroko, P.O. Box 1034, Papua New Guinea.

University of Papua New Guinea, Faculty of Medicine, P.O. Box 5623, Boroko, Papua New Guinea.

PERU

Ministerio de Salud Publica, Asistencia Social, Area de Puno, Avenida Salaverry, Lima, Peru.

PHILIPPINES

Community Development Research Council, University of the Philippines, Dilimar, Quezon City, Philippines.

Department of Health & The Institute of Public Health, University of Philippines, Manila, Philippines.

Entrepreneurial Development Centre Inc., Far East Building, Buendia Avenue, Cor. Pasong Tamo, Makati, Rizal, Philippines.

Family Planning Organization of the Philippines, P.O. Box 1279, Manila, Philippines.

International Institute of Rural Reconstruction, Silang, Cavite, Philippines.

International Secretariat for Volunteer Service (ISVS), Asian Regional Office, 503 B. Jalandoni Building, 1444 A. Madine Street, Ermita, Manila, Philippines.

Nutrition Department, University of the Philippines, Dilimar, Quezon City, Philippines.

Rural Missionaries of the Philippines. 2215 Pedro Gil, Sta Ana, Manila, Philippines.

Silliman University Medical Centre, P.O. Box 49, Dumaguete City, Philippines.

World Health Organization Regional Office for the Western Pacific, P.O. Box 2932, 12115 Manila, Philippines.

PUERTO RICO

Brethren Service Project, P.O. Box 23, Castaner, Puerto Rico 00631.

RHODESIA

Family Planning Association of Rhodesia, P.O. Box St 22, Southerton, Salisbury, Rhodesia.

University of Rhodesia, Department of Medicine, Harari Central Hospital, P.O. Box St 14, Southerton, Salisbury, Rhodesia.

SIERRA LEONE

Methodist Training Centre, Nixon Memorial Hospital, Segbwema, Sierra Leone.

SOLOMON ISLANDS

Director of Medical Services, Medical Department, P.O. Box G 349, Honiara, Solomon Islands.

Gizo Hospital, Medical Department, Western District, Solomon Islands.

Health Department, Medical Services Division, Guadalcanal, Solomon Islands.

SOMALIA

Ministry of Health, Mogadishu, Somalia.

SOUTH AFRICA

All Saints Hospital, P.O. All Saints, Transkei.

Department of Obstetrics & Gynaecology, Medical School, P.O. Box 17039, Congella, Durban 4013, Natal, South Africa.

Department of Paediatrics & Child Health, University of Cape Town, Rondebosch, Cape Town, South Africa.

SUDAN

University of Khartoum, Department of Paediatrics and Child Health, Faculty of Medicine, P.O. Box 102, Khartoum, Democratic Republic of the Sudan.

SWEDEN

The Dag Hammarskjöld Foundation, Dag Hammarskjöld Centre, Ovre Slottsgatan 2, S-752 20, Uppsala, Sweden.

Department of Paediatrics, University Hospital, Linkoping, Sweden.

Department of Social Medicine, Scandinavian School of Public Health, Gothenburg, Sweden.

Goteburg Universitet, Medicinsk-Kemiska Instutionen Medicinaregatan 9, Goteburg, Sweden.

SWITZERLAND

Christian Medical Commission, World Council of Churches, 150 Route de Ferney, 1211 Geneva 20, Switzerland.

International Labour Office, CH 1211 Geneva 22, Switzerland.

League of Red Cross Societies, P.O. Box 276, 1211 Geneva 19, Switzerland.

Lutheran World Service, P.O. Box 66, Route de Ferney 150, 1211 Geneva, Switzerland.

REMAHA, World Health Organization, 1211 Geneva 27, Switzerland.

Swiss Tropical Institute, Socinstrasse 57, 4051 Basle, Switzerland.
UNICEF—Regional Office for Europe & North Africa, Palais des Nations, CH 1211 Geneva 10, Switzerland.
World Health Organization (WHO), 1211 Geneva 27, Switzerland.

TANZANIA

East Africa Literature Bureau, P.O. Box 1408, Dar es Salaam, Tanzania.

East African Institute for Medical Research, P.O. Box 1462, Mwanza, Tanzania.

Institute of Adult Education, University of Dar es Salaam, P.O. Box 35091, Dar es Salaam, Tanzania.

Medical Assistants' Training Centre, Bumbuli, Tanzania.

Ministry of Health, Tanzania Consultant Hospitals, Kilimanjaro Christian Medical Centre, Private Bag, Moshi, Tanzania.

Ministry of Health & Social Welfare, P.O. Box 9383, Dar es Salaam, Tanzania.

Tanzania Christian Medical Association, P.O. Box 9433, Dar es Salaam, Tanzania.

Tanzania Food & Nutrition Centre, P.O. Box 9383, Dar es Salaam, Tanzania.

University of Dar es Salaam, Faculty of Medicine, P.O. Box 20693, Dar es Salaam, Tanzania.

THAILAND

Chonburi Health Training Centre, Division of Health Training Office, Ministry of Public Health, Bangkok, Thailand.

Community Based Family Planning Services (CBFPS), 8 Sukhmvit Soi 12, Bangkok, Thailand.

Ministry of Public Health, Samsen Road, Bangkok, Thailand.

Thai National Documentation Centre, Applied Scientific Research Corporation of Thailand, Bang Khen, Bangkok 9, Thailand.

UNICEF—Regional Office for East Asia & Pakistan, P.O. Box 2-154, Bangkok, Thailand.

UGANDA

East Africa Literature Bureau, P.O. Box 1317, Kampala, Uganda.

Medical Assistants Training School, Mbale, Uganda.

104

Ministry of Health, P.O. Box 16394, Mandegeya, Kampala, Uganda.

M.R.C. Child Nutrition Unit, Mulago Hospital, P.O. Box 7051, Kampala, Uganda.

UNITED KINGDOM

African Studies Group, King's College, Aberdeen University, Scotland, U.K.

Appropriate Health Resources and Technologies Action Group (AHRTAG), 85 Marylebone High Street, London W1M 3DE, U.K.

Baptist Missionary Society, 93–97 Gloucester Place, London W1H 1AA, U.K.

British Council, 65 Davies Street, London W1Y 2AA, U.K.

British Medical Association, Department of Audio Visual Communication, Tavistock Square, London WC1H 9JP, U.K.

British Red Cross Society, 9 Grosvenor Crescent, London SW1, U.K.

Catholic Institute for International Relations, 1 Cambridge Terrace, London NW1, U.K.

Centre for Educational Development Overseas (CEDO), Tavistock House, South Entrance D, Tavistock Square, London WC1, U.K.

Ciba Foundation, 41 Portland Place, London W1N 4BN, U.K.

Commonwealth Foundation, Marlborough House, Pall Mall, London SW1, U.K.

Conference of Missionary Societies in Great Britain & Ireland, Edinburgh House, 2 Eaton Gate, London SW1W 9BL, U.K.

Department of Social Science, London School of Economics, Houghton Street, Aldwych, London WC2, U.K.

Institute of Child Health, 30 Guilford Street, London WC1N 1EH, U.K.

Institute of Development Studies, University of Sussex, Andrew Cohen Building, Falmer, Brighton, Sussex BN1 9RE, U.K.

Intermediate Technology Development Group (ITDG), 9 King Street, London WC2E 8HN, U.K.

Intermediate Technology Publications Ltd, 9 King Street, London WC2E 8HN, U.K.

International Planned Parenthood Federation (IPPF), 18–20 Lower Regent Street, London SW1Y 4PW, U.K.

The Leprosy Mission, 50 Portland Place, London W1, U.K.

Leprosy Study Centre, 57a Wimpole Street, London W1, U.K.

105

Liverpool School of Tropical Medicine, University of Liverpool, Department of Tropical Community Health, Pembroke Place, Liverpool L3 5QA, U.K.

London School of Hygiene & Tropical Medicine, Keppel Street, Gower Street, London WC1E 7HT, U.K.

London Technical Group, 85 Marylebone High Street, London W1M 3DE, U.K.

Medical Architecture Research Unit, Northern Polytechnic, Holloway Road, London N7, U.K.

Medical Missionary Association, 6 Cannonbury Place, London N1 2NJ, U.K.

Medical Recording Service Foundation, Royal College of General Practitioners, Kitts Croft, Writtle, Chelmsford CM1 3EH, U.K.

The National Fund for Research into Crippling Diseases, Vincent House, Vincent Square, London SW1, U.K.

Office of Health Economics, 130 Regent Street, London W1R 6DD, U.K.

Oxfam, 274 Banbury Road, Oxford OX2 7DZ, U.K.

Ross Institute, London School of Hygiene & Tropical Medicine, Keppel Street, Gower Street, London WC1E 7HT, U.K.

Rural Communications Services, 64 West Street, South Petherton, Somerset, U.K.

School for Dental Auxiliaries, New Cross Hospital, Avonley Road, London SE14 5ER, U.K.

School of Medicine, University of Newcastle, Newcastle upon Tyne, NE1 7RU, U.K.

St John Ambulance Association, Priory House, St. John's Gate, Clerkenwell, London EC1M 4DA, U.K.

Survival International, 36 Craven Street, London WC2, U.K.

Teaching Aids at Low Cost (TALC), Institute of Child Health, 30 Guilford Street, London WC1N 1EH, U.K.

Third World Publications, 67 College Road, Birmingham B13 9LR, U.K.

University of Aberdeen, Department of Surgery, University Medical Buildings, Foresterhill, Aberdeen AB9 2ZD, U.K.

University of Edinburgh, Department of Nursing Studies, Nursing Research Unit, 12 Buccleuch Place, Edinburgh EH8 9JT, U.K.

University of Glasgow, Social Paediatric & Obstetric Research Unit, Department of Child Health & Obstetrics, 23 Montrose Street, Glasgow G1 1RN, U.K.

University of Manchester, Department of Social & Preventive

106

Medicine, Clinical Sciences Building, York Place, Manchester M13 0JJ, U.K.

University of Nottingham, Department of Community Health, University of Nottingham Medical School, University Park, Nottingham NG7 2RD, U.K.

War on Want, 467 Caledonian Road, London N7 9BE, U.K.

Wellcome Museum of Medical Science, P.O. Box 129, 183 Euston Road, London NW1 2BP, U.K.

Wellcome Trust, 1 Park Square West, London NW1 4LJ, U.K.

UNITED STATES OF AMERICA

African Inland Mission, P.O. Box 178, Pearl River, NY 10965, U.S.A.

Aid for International Development (AID), Department of State, 320 Twenty-first Street N.W., Washington, D.C. 20523, U.S.A.

American Association of Medical Assistants Inc., 200 East Ohio Street, Chicago, Illinois 60611, U.S.A.

American Friends Service Committee, Latin America Program, 160 No. Fifteenth Street, Philadelphia, Penna 19102, U.S.A.

American Journal of Chinese Medicine, now called Comparative Medicine East & West, P.O. Box 555, Garden City, New York, NY 11530, U.S.A.

American Leprosy Missions Inc., 297 Park Avenue South, New York, NY 10010, U.S.A.

American Public Health Association, 1015 Eighteenth Street, N.W., Washington, D.C. 20036, U.S.A.

Association of Schools of Allied Health Professions, 1 Dupont Circle, Washington, D.C. 20036, U.S.A.

Behrhorst Clinic Foundation Inc., 50 Haven Avenue, New York, NY 10032, U.S.A.

Clinica de Salubridad de Campesinos, 116 "K" Street, P.O. Box 1279, Brawley, California 92227, U.S.A.

Commonwealth of Massachusetts, Department of Public Health, 600 Washington Street, Boston 02111, U.S.A.

Community Systems Foundation, 1130 Hill Street, Ann Arbor, Michigan 48104, U.S.A.

Department of Epidemiology & Public Health, Yale University of Medicine, 60 College Street, New Haven, Connecticut 06510, U.S.A.

Department of Health, Education & Welfare (DHEW), Office of

International Health, Division of Professional Resources, 330 Independence Avenue, S.W., Washington, D.C. 20201, U.S.A.

Department of Health, Education & Welfare, Public Health Service, National Institution of Health, Bethesda, Maryland 20014, U.S.A.

Department of Health, Education & Welfare, Division of Indian Health, Juneau, Alaska, U.S.A.

Department of Medicine, Beth Israel Hospital, 330 Brookline Avenue, Boston, Mass. 12215, U.S.A.

Development Project Management Center, US Department of Agriculture, Department of State, 320 Twenty-first Street, N.W., Washington, D.C. 20523, U.S.A.

Direct Relief Foundation, 27 East Canon Perdido Street, Santa Barbara, California 93101, U.S.A.

East-West Communication Institute, 1777 East-West Road, Honolulu, Hawaii 96822, U.S.A.

Family Health Inc., 136 South Roman Street, New Orleans, Louisiana 70112, U.S.A.

Harvard School of Public Health, 55 Shattuck Street, Boston, Massachusetts 02115, U.S.A.

The Hesperian Foundation, P.O. Box1692, Palo Alto, California 94302, U.S.A.

Institute for Health Research, 2150 Shattuck Avenue, Berkeley, California 94704, U.S.A.

International Association for Prevention of Blindness, Suite 280, 1013 Bishop Street, Honolulu, Hawaii 96813, U.S.A.

The International Childbirth Education Association Inc., Box 22, Hillside, New Jersey 07205, U.S.A.

International Institute of Rural Reconstruction, U.S. Office, 1775 Broadway, New York, NY 10019, U.S.A.

International Medical & Research Foundation, Warrenton, Virginia, U.S.A.

International Task Force on World Health Manpower, c/o Medical Tribune, 110 East Fifty-ninth Street, New York, NY 10022, U.S.A.

John E. Fogarty International Center for Advanced Study in the Health Sciences, National Institutes of Health, Bethesda, Maryland, Md. 20014, U.S.A.

John Hopkins University, School of Hygiene & Public Health, Department of International Health, 615 North Wolfe Street, Baltimore, Maryland 21205, U.S.A.

Josiah Macy Foundation, 1 Rockefeller Foundation, New York, NY 10020, U.S.A.

108

Medex Program, Dartmouth Medical School, Nugget Arcade, P.O. Box 146, Hanover, New Hampshire 03755, U.S.A.

Medex Program, University of Hawaii, School of Medicine, 1960 East-West Road, Honolulu, Hawaii 96822, U.S.A.

Medical Assistance Programs (MAP), Box 50, Wheaton, Illinois, U.S.A.

The National Center for Health Statistics, 5600 Fischer Lane, Rockville, Maryland 20852, U.S.A.

National Tuberculosis & Respiratory Disease Association, 1740 Broadway, New York, NY 10019, U.S.A.

New Health Careers Demonstration Project, Institute for Health Research, Berkeley, California, U.S.A.

New York Academy of Medicine, 2 East 103rd Street, New York, NY 10029, U.S.A.

Northern University College of Pharmacy & Allied Health Professions, Physician Assistant Program, Robinson Hall 202, North-eastern University, Boston, Mass. 02115, U.S.A.

Office of Health Affairs, Office of Economic Opportunity, 100 McAlister Street, 26th Floor, San Francisco, California 94102, U.S.A.

Office of International Health Programs, Harvard School of Public Health, 677 Huntingdon Avenue, Boston, Massachusetts, U.S.A.

Pan American Health Organization (PAHO), 52–5 Twenty-third Street, N.W., Washington, D.C. 20037, U.S.A.

The People to People Health Foundation (Project Hope), 2233 Wisconsin Avenue, N.W., Washington, D.C. 20007, U.S.A.

Planned Parenthood World Population, 515 Madison Avenue, New York, U.S.A.

The Population Council, 1 Dag Hammarskjöld Plaza, New York, NY 10017, U.S.A.

Population Crisis Committee, 1835 K. Street, N.W., Washington, D.C. 20006, U.S.A.

Project Concern, 3802 Houston Street, San Diego, California 92110, U.S.A.

Protein Advisory Group, c/o United Nations, U.N. Plaza, New York, NY 10017, U.S.A.

Research Corporation, 505 Lexington Avenue, New York, NY 10017, U.S.A.

School of Public Health, University of California, Los Angeles, California 90024, U.S.A.

Sound Health Corporation, P.O. Box 609, Nome, Alaska 99762, U.S.A.

State University of New York, Downstate Medical Center, Department of Obstetrics & Gynaecology, 450 Clarkson Avenue, Brooklyn, NY 11203, U.S.A.

Student Health Program for Migrant Farmworkers, c/o University of Colorado Medical Center, 4200 East 9th Avenue, Denver, COLO 80220, U.S.A.

United States National Health Service Corps, Department of Health, Education & Welfare, Public Health Service, Health Services & Mental Health Administration, Rockville, Maryland 20852, U.S.A.

University of California, Danfa Comprehensive Rural Health & Family Planning Project, School of Public Health, University of California, Los Angeles, California 90024, U.S.A.

University of California Extension, Maternal and Child Health Project, Santa Cruz, California 95060, U.S.A.

University of Michigan, Department of Medical Care Organization, School of Public Health, Ann Arbor, Michigan 48104, U.S.A.

University of North Carolina, School of Medicine, Self-Instructional Materials Project, Chapel Hill, North Carolina 27514, U.S.A.

University of Pennsylvania, School of Medicine, Department of Community Medicine, 36th and Hamilton Walk, Philadelphia, Penn. 19104, U.S.A.

Volunteers in Technical Assistance (VITA), 3706 Rhode Island Avenue, Mount Rainier, Maryland 20822, U.S.A.

World Education, 1414 Avenue of the Americas, New York, NY 10019, U.S.A.

World Health Organization Regional Office for the Americas, Pan American Sanitary Bureau, 525, 23rd Street, N.W., Washington, D.C. 20037, U.S.A.

World Neighbours, 5116 North Portland Avenue, Oklahoma City, Oklahoma 73112, U.S.A.

Yale University School of Medicine, Trauma Program, Department of Surgery, 333 Cedar Street, New Haven, Connecticut 06510, U.S.A.

Yukon Kuskokim Health Corporation, P.O. Box 536, Ethel, Alaska 99559, U.S.A.

VENEZUELA

Centro Medico Docente la Trinidad, 50 Piso Oficina 502, Avedida Andres Bello, Apartado Postal 50676, Caracas 105, Venezuela.

110

Department de Medicina Preventiva y Social, Universidad de los Andes, Apartado 185, Merida, Venezuela.

Instituto Nacional de Dermatologia, Providencia a San Nicolas, San Jose, Caracas, Venezuela.

Laboratorio Para Estudios Sobre Malaria Edificio Anexo, Instituto Nacional de Higiene Ciudad Universitaria, Apartado Postal No. 4417, Caracas 101, Venezuela.

Ministerio de Sanidad y Asistencia Social, Oficina de Publicaciónes, Biblioteca y Archivo, Caracas, Venezuela.

Universidad Simon Bolivar, Sartenejas, Baruta, Edo. Miranda-Apartado Postal 5354, Caracas, Venezuela.

WEST INDIES

Trinidad Regional Virus Laboratory, 16–18 Jamaica Boulevard, P.O. Box 164, Federation Park, St. Clair, West Indies.

University of the West Indies, Department of Social & Preventive Medicine, Mona, Kingston 7, Jamaica, West Indies.

YEMEN

Turba Rural Health Project, Hugariah District, Yemen Arab Republic.

ZAIRE

Bureau d'Etudes et de Recherches pour la Promotion de la Santé, B.P. 1977, Kangu-Mayombe, Zaire.

Centre Protestant d'Editions et de Diffusion (CEDI), B.P. 123, Kinshasa, Zaire.

Centre Medical de Kisantu, Zone Rurale, B.P. 46, Inkisi, Zaire.

L'Ecole d'Infirmiers Auxiliaires, Hôpital de Pimu, B.P. 23, Lisala, Equateur, Zaire.

L'Ecole d'Infirmiers Auxiliaires, B.P. 20, Dungu via Isiro, Haut Zaire, Zaire.

Formation Medicale de Mikalayi, B.P. 70, Mikalayi, Kananga, Kasai Occidental, Zaire.

Institut Medical Evangelique, B.P. 68, Kimpese, Bas Zaire, Zaire.

Medical Auxiliary Training School, CBZO, Vanga, B.P. 4728, Kinshasa 2, Zaire.

ZAMBIA

Medical Assistants Training School, Chainama Hills, P.O. Box 3191, Lusaka, Zambia.

Ministry of Health, P.O. Box 174, Lusaka, Zambia.

National Food & Nutrition Commission, P.O. Box 2669, Lusaka, Zambia.

Journals referred to in the Bibliography

AFYA
African Medical & Research
Foundation
P.O. Box 30125
Nairobi
Kenya

American Journal of Clinical Nutrition
9650 Rockville Pike
Bethesda
Maryland 20014
U.S.A.

American Journal of Public Health
American Public Health
Association
1015 18th Street, N.W.
Washington, D.C. 20036
U.S.A.

Appropriate Technology
9 King Street
London WC2E 8HN
U.K.

British Dental Journal
64 Wimpole Street
London W1M 8AL
U.K.

British Journal of Nutrition
Cambridge University Press
200 Euston Road
London NW1 2DB
U.K.

British Medical Journal
B.M.A. House
Tavistock Square
London WC1
U.K.

Bulletin of the New York Academy
New York Academy of
Medicine
2 East 103rd Street
New York, NY 10029
U.S.A.

Bulletin Penelitian Kesehatan
Health Studies in Indonesia
Lembaga Research Kesehatan
Nasional
Division of Publications &
Libraries
Department of Health
Jl Percetaken Negara No. 1
Jakarta
Indonesia

Cajanus
Carribean Food & Nutrition
Institute
P.O. Box 140
Kingston 7
Jamaica

Carnet de L'Enfance—
Assignment Children
UNICEF
Palais Wilson
Case postale 11
1211 Geneva 14
Switzerland

Community Development Journal
Oxford University Press
Press Road
Neasden
London NW10 0DD
U.K.

Contact
Christian Medical Commission
World Council of Churches
150 Route de Ferney
1211 Geneva 20
Switzerland

Courier of the International
Children's Centre
Chateau de Longchamp
Bois de Boulogne
75 Paris 16e
France

Ecodevelopment News
54 Boulevard Raspail
Bureau 309
75270 Paris Cedex 06
France

Educational Development
International
Development Education
Exchange
Action for Development
Food and Agriculture
Organization
00100 Rome
Italy

English Language Teaching
Journal
Oxford University Press
Press Road
Neasden
London NW10 0DD
U.K.

IDRC Reports
Box 8500
Ottawa
Canada K1G 3H9

International Journal of
Contemporary Sociology
Rakesh Marg
Pili Kothi
G. T. Road
Ghaziabad, U.P.
India

Israel Journal of Medical
Science
Israel Medical Association
Box 1435
Jerusalem
Israel

Journal of American Medical
Association
American Medical Association
535 North Deasborn Street
Chicago
Illinois 60610
U.S.A.

Journal of Development Studies
67 Great Russell Street
London WC1B 3BT
U.K.

Journal of Eastern Medicine
Hamdard Foundation
Nazimabad
Karachi 18
Pakistan

Journal of Medical & Dental
Association
Mahalapye
Botswana

**Journal of Tropical Paediatrics
& Environmental Child Health**
2 Drayson Mews
Kensington
London W8
U.K.

**League for International Food
Education Newsletter**
1126 16th Street, N.W.
Room 404
Washington, D.C. 20036
U.S.A.

The Lancet
7 Adam Street
Adelphi
London WC2
U.K.

Medico Friend Circle
21 Nirman Society
Vadodara 390 005
Gujarat
India

**New England Journal of
Medicine**
Massachusetts Medical Society
10 Shattuck Street
Boston
Massachusetts 02115
U.S.A.

New Scientist
King's Reach Tower
Stamford Street
London SE1
U.K.

Nutrition Newsletter
Food Policy & Nutrition
Division
Food & Agriculture
Organization
Via delle Terme di Caracalla
00100 Rome
Italy

PAG Bulletin
Room 555
866 United Nations Plaza
New York, NY 10017
U.S.A.

Pan American Health
Pan American Health
Organization
525, 23rd Street, N.W.
Washington, D.C. 20037
U.S.A.

People Magazine
IPPF Publications
18–20 Lower Regent Street
London SW1Y 4PW
U.K.

**Rocky Mountain Medical
Journal**
Colorado Medical Society
1601 E 19th Avenue
Denver CO 80218
U.S.A.

Salubritas
American Public Health
Association
International Health Programs
1015 18th Street, N.W.
Washington, D.C. 20036
U.S.A.

**Social Science & Medicine
Journal**
Maxwell House
Fairview Park
New York, NY 10523
U.S.A.

South African Medical Journal
P.O. Box 643
Capetown 8000
South Africa

South East Asian Journal of Tropical Medicine & Public Health
420 6 Rajvithi Road
Bangkok 4
Thailand

Tropical Doctor
Royal Society of Medicine
Chandos House
2 Queen Anne Street
London W1M 0BR
U.K.

Tropical & Geographical Medicine
De Erven Bohn B.V.
Amsterdam
The Netherlands

WHO Chronicle
World Health Organization
Avenue Appia
1211 Geneva 27
Switzerland

World Education
1414 Avenue of the Americas
New York, NY 10019
U.S.A.

World Health
World Health Organization
Avenue Appia
1211 Geneva 27
Switzerland

World Hospitals
International Hospital
Federation
24 Nutford Place
London W1
U.K.

World Medical Journal
World Medical Association
10 Columbus Circle
New York, NY 10019
U.S.A.

World Medicine
Clareville House
26–27 Oxenden Street
London SW1Y 4EL
U.K.

World Review of Nutrition & Dietetics
Arnhold-Bocklin-Str. 25
4011 Basel
Switzerland

Publishers Referred to in the Bibliography

African Medical & Research Foundation
P.O. Box 30125
Nairobi
Kenya

African Studies Group
King's College
Aberdeen University
Scotland
U.K.

All Africa Leprosy & Rehabilitation Training Centre (ALERT)
P.O. Box 165
Addis Ababa
Ethiopia

American Leprosy Missions Inc.
297 Park Avenue South
New York, NY 10010
U.S.A.

Appleton Century-Crofts
440 Park Avenue South
New York, NY 10016
U.S.A.

Asia Publishing House
Calicut Street
Bombay
India.

British Hospitals Export Council
24 Nutford Place
London W1
U.K.

British Red Cross Society
9 Grosvenor Crescent
London SW1
U.K.

Bureau d'Etudes et de Recherches pour la Promotion de la Santé
B.P. 1977
Kangu-Mayombe
Zaire

Butterworths
Borough Green
Sevenoaks
Kent
U.K.

Canadian Universities Service Overseas (CUSO)
151 Slater Street
Ottawa
Ontario, K1P5H5
Canada

The Caribbean Institute on Mental Retardation and Development Disabilities
2D Suthermere Road
Kingston
Jamaica

117

Catholic Institute for
International Relations
1 Cambridge Terrace
London NW1
U.K.

Centre International de
L'Enfance
Chateau de Longchamp
Bois de Boulogne
75016 Paris
France

Centre Medical de Kisantu
Zone Rurale
B.P. 46
Inkisi
Zaire

Chonburi Health Training
Centre
Division of Health Training
Office
Ministry of Public Health
Bangkok
Thailand

Christian Conference of Asia
c/o Hong Kong Christian
Council
57 Peking Road 4/F
Kowloon
Hong Kong

Christian Council of Nigeria
Ikot Ibritam
PMB 38
Abak
South Eastern States
Nigeria

Christian Medical Association of
India
Christian Council Lodge
Nagpur 440 001
Madya Pradesh
India

Christian Medical Commission
World Council of Churches
150 Route de Ferney
1211 Geneva 20
Switzerland

Churchill Livingstone
33 Montgomery Street
Edinburgh EH7 5JX
Scotland
U.K.

Ciba Foundation
41 Portland Place
London W1N 4BN
U.K.

Clausen Publications
115 St. Mary's Road
Weybridge
Surrey
U.K.

Commonwealth Foundation
Marlborough House,
Pall Mall
London SW1Y 5HX
U.K.

Commonwealth Secretariat
Marlborough House
Pall Mall
London SW1Y 5HX
U.K.

Community Systems Foundation
1130 Hill Street
Ann Arbor
Michigan 48104
U.S.A.

Conference of Missionary
Societies in Great Britain &
Ireland
Edinburgh House
2 Eaton Gate
London SW1W 9BL
U.K.

Cornell University Press
124 Roberts Place
Ithaca
New York, NY 14850
U.S.A.

The Dag Hammarskjöld
Foundation
Dag Hammarskjöld Centre
Ovre Slottsgatan 2
S-752 20
Uppsala
Sweden

Delmar Publications
Mountainview Avenue
Albany, NY 12205
U.S.A.

Department of Extension &
Training
Ministry of Agriculture &
Natural Resources
Lilongwe
Malawi

Department of Health & Welfare
Division of Indian Health
Juneau
Alaska
U.S.A.

Department of Health Services
Ministry of Health
Kathmandu
Nepal

Department of National Health
& Welfare
Publications Department
Brooke-Claxton Building
Ottawa K1A 0K9
Canada

Department of Public Health
Paramedical College
P.O. Box 2033
Yomba, Madang
Papua New Guinea

Department of Social Medicine
Scandinavian School of Public
Health
Gothenburg
Sweden

Directorate General of
Community Health
Ministry of Health
Parapattan 10
Jakarta
Indonesia

East Africa Literature Bureau
P.O. Box 3002, Nairobi, Kenya
P.O. Box 1408, Dar es Salaam,
Tanzania
P.O. Box 1317, Kampala,
Uganda

East-West Communication
Institute
1777 East-West Road
Honolulu
Hawaii 96822
U.S.A.

Editions Saint Paul
Issy-les-Moulineaux
Limete
Kinshasa
Zaire

Editorial Pax-Maxico
Libreria Carlos Cesarman, S.A.
Apartado Postal 45-009
Mexico, D.F.
Mexico

B. Edsall & Co
26 Eccleston Square
London SW1V 1PF
U.K.

Edward Arnold Ltd
125 Hill Street
London W1
U.K.

119

El Ateneo Pedro Garcia
S.A.L.E.
1 Florida 340
Buenos Aires
Argentina

Emmanuel Hospitals Association
808/92 Nehru Place
New Delhi 110 024
India

The English Universities Press Ltd, now called **Hodder & Stoughton Ltd.**
P.O. Box 6
Mill Road
Dunton Green
Sevenoaks
Kent TN13 2XX
U.K.

Family Planning Association of Rhodesia
P.O. Box ST 220
Southerton
Salisbury
Rhodesia

Family Planning Organisation of the Philippines
P.O. Box 1279
Manila
Philippines

Fearon Publications
Palo Alto
California 94022
U.S.A.

Food & Agriculture Organization (FAO)
Publications Division
Via delle Terme di Caracalla
00100 Rome
Italy

Gonashasthaya Kendra
P.O. Nayarhat
District Dacca
Bangladesh

Goteborg Universite
Medicinsk-Kemiska
Institutionen
Medicinaregatan 9
Goteburg
Sweden

The Government Printer
Zomba
Malawi

Hamdard National Foundation
Nazimabad
Karachi 18
Pakistan

Heinemann Medical Books Ltd.
23 Bedford Square
London WC1
U.K.

The Hesperian Foundation
P.O. Box 1692
Palo Alto
California 94302
U.S.A.

IBEG Ltd.
2 Brook Street
London W1Y 1AA
U.K.

Institut Penyelidikan Perubatan
International Centre for
Medical Research
University of California
Kuala Lumpur
Malaysia

Institute of Adult Education
University of Dar es Salaam
P.O. Box 35091
Dar es Salaam
Tanzania

Institute of Development Studies
University of Sussex
Andrew Cohen Building
Falmer
Brighton
Sussex BN1 9RE
U.K.

Intermediate Technology
Publications Ltd.
9 King Street
London WC2E 8HN
U.K.

The International Childbirth
Education Association Inc.
Box 22
Hillside
New Jersey 07205
U.S.A.

International Development
Research Centre
P.O. Box 8500
Ottawa K1G 3H9
Canada

International Labour
Organisation
CH-1211 Geneva 22
Switzerland

International Medical &
Research Foundation
Warrenton
Virginia
U.S.A.

International Secretariat for
Volunteer Service
Asian Regional Office
503 B. Jaladoni Building
1444 A. Madine Street
Ermita
Manila
Philippines

John E. Fogarty International
Centre for Advanced Study in the
Health Sciences
National Institutes of Health
Bethesda
Maryland, Md. 20014
U.S.A.

John Wiley & Sons Ltd
Baffins Lane
Chichester
Sussex PO19 1UD
U.K.

Johns Hopkins Press
Baltimore, MD 21218
U.S.A.

Josiah Macy Foundation
1 Rockefeller Foundation
New York, NY 10020
U.S.A.

Khartoum University Press
P.O. Box 321
Khartoum
Sudan

Lange Medical Publications
Los Altos
California 94022
U.S.A.

League of Red Cross Societies
P.O. Box 276
1211 Geneva 19
Switzerland

Lembaga Kesehatan Nasional
Jl. Perceraken Negara No.1
Indonesia

The Leprosy Mission
50 Portland Place
London W1
U.K.

Little, Brown & Co.
34 Beacon Street
Boston, MA 02106
U.S.A.

Lloyd Luke Ltd.
49 Newman Street
London W1
U.K.

Lutheran World Service
P.O. Box 66
Route de Ferney 150
1211 Geneva
Switzerland

Lutterworth Press
Luke House
Farnham Road
Guildford
Surrey GU1 4XD
U.K.

Macmillan & Co. Ltd.
4 Little Essex Street
London WC2
U.K.

Macmillan International Ltd.
P.O. Box 264
Yaba
Lagos
Nigeria

Marquette University Press
1311 W. Wisconsin Avenue
Milwaukee
Wisconsin 53233
U.S.A.

McGraw Hill International Publications
34 Dover Street
London W1
U.K.
also 348 Jalan Boon Lay
Jurong
Singapore 22

Medical Assistance Programmes (MAP)
Box 50
Wheaton
Illinois
U.S.A.

Medical Assistants Training School
Chainama Hills
P.O. Box 3191
Lusaka
Zambia

Medical Auxiliaries Training School
Sudan Interior Mission
Jos
Nigeria

Medical Missionary Association
6 Cannonbury Place
London N1 2NJ
U.K.

Medico Friends Circle
21 Nirman Society
Vadodara 390 005
Gujarat
India

Ministerio de Salud Publica
Division de Atención Medica
Bogota D.E.
Colombia

Ministerio de Salud Publica Asistencia Social
Area de Puno
Avenida Salaverry
Lima
Peru

Ministry of Health
Jalan Young
Kuala Lumpur
Malaysia

Ministry of Health & Family
Welfare
Nirman Bhavan
New Delhi 110 001
India

Ministry of Health and Social
Welfare
P.O. Box 9383
Dar es Salaam
Tanzania

C. V. Mosby Co. Ltd.
11830 Westline Industrial Drive
St. Louis, MO 63141
U.S.A.

M.R.C. Child Nutrition Unit
Mulago Hospital
Box 7051
Kampala
Uganda

The National Food & Nutrition
Commission
P.O. Box 2669
Lusaka
Zambia

The National Fund for Research
into Crippling Diseases
Vincent House
Vincent Square
London SW1
U.K.

National Institute of Health &
Family Welfare
L17 Green Park
New Delhi 110 016
India

National Printing Co. Ltd.
P.O. Box 2320
Dar es Salaam
Tanzania

Near East Ecumenical
Committee for Palestine
Refugees
P.O. Box 4047
Nicosia
Cyprus

The Nestlé Company (Australia)
17 Foveaux Street
Sydney
New South Wales
Australia

Nursing Education Division
Department of Public Health
P.O. Box 2084
Konedobu
Papua New Guinea

OECD Development Centre
94 rue Chardon-Lagache
75016 Paris
France

Office of Health Affairs
Office of Economic Opportunity
100 McAlister Street
26th Floor
San Francisco
California 94102
U.S.A.

Office of Health Economics
130 Regent Street
London W1R 6DD
U.K.

Oxfam
274 Banbury Road
Oxford OX2 7DZ
U.K.

Oxford Medical Publications
Ely House
London W1
U.K.

Oxford University Press
P.O. Box 72532
Nairobi
Kenya
also 37 Dover Street
London W1
U.K.

**Pan American Health
Organization (PAHO)**
52–5 23rd Street, N.W.,
Washington, D.C. 20037
U.S.A.

Paramedical College
P.O. Box 2033
Yomba
Madang
Papua New Guinea

**The People to People Health
Foundation Inc. (Project Hope)**
2233 Wisconsin Avenue, N.W.
Washington, D.C. 20007
U.S.A.

**Planned Parenthood World
Population**
515 Madison Avenue
New York
U.S.A.

Population Crisis Committee
1835 K. Street, N.W.
Washington, D.C. 20006
U.S.A.

Port Moresby General Hospital
Boroko
P.O. Box 1034
Papua New Guinea

Praeger Publishers
111 Fourth Avenue
New York, NY 10003
U.S.A.

**Prince Leopold Institute of
Tropical Medicine**
Nationalestraat 155
B-2000 Antwerp
Belgium

Protein Advisory Group
United Nations
United Nations Plaza
New York, NY 10017
U.S.A.

Publishing Sciences Group Inc.
Acton
Massachussetts
U.S.A.

REMAHA
World Health Organization
1211 Geneva 27
Switzerland

Ross Institute
London School of Hygiene &
Tropical Medicine
Keppel Street
London WC1E 7HT
U.K.

Royal Tropical Institute
Department of Tropical Hygiene
63 Mauritskade
Amsterdam-Oost
The Netherlands

124

Rural Communications Services
64 West Street
South Petherton
Somerset
U.K.

Rural Health Research Centre
Narngwal
District Ludhiana
Punjab
India

Rural Missionaries of the Philippines
2215 Pedro Gil
Sta Ana
Manila
Philippines

Shanta Bhawan Hospital
Box 252
Kathmandu
Nepal

Silliman University Medical Centre
P.O. Box 49
Dumaguete City
Philippines

Social Science & Medicine Journals Department
Maxwell House
Fairview Park
New York NY 10523
U.S.A.

St. John Ambulance Association
Priory House
St. John's Gate
Clerkenwell
London EC1M 4DA
U.K.

TALC see Teaching Aids at Low Cost

Tanzania Publishing House
Box 2138
Dar es Salaam
Tanzania

Teaching Aids at Low Cost (TALC)
Institute of Child Health
30 Guilford Street
London WC1N 1EH
U.K.

Third World Publications
67 College Road
Birmingham B13 9LR
U.K.

Tri-Med Books
5 Tudor Cottage
Lovers Walk
Finchley
London N3 1JH
U.K.

UNICEF
United Nations Plaza
New York, NY 10007
U.S.A.

UNICEF—East Africa
P.O. Box 44145
Nairobi
Kenya

UNICEF—South Central Asia
11 Jor Bagh
New Delhi 110 003
India

University of Dar es Salaam
P.O. Box 35091
Dar es Salaam
Tanzania

125

University of London
Queen Elizabeth College
Campden Hill Road
London W8
U.K.

University of West Indies
Department of Social &
Preventive Medicine
Mona, Kingston
7 Jamaica

Van den Berghs & Jurgens Ltd.
Sussex House
Burgess Hill
West Sussex RH15 9AW
U.K.

Voluntary Health Association of India
C14 Community Centre
Safdarjung Development Area
New Delhi 110 016
India

Volunteers in Technical Assistance (VITA)
3706 Rhode Island Avenue
Mount Rainier
Maryland 20822
U.S.A.

Vuga Press
P.O. Box 25
Soni
Tanzania

War on Want
467 Caledonian Road
London N7 9BE
U.K.

World Education
1414 Avenue of the Americas
New York, NY 10019
U.S.A.

World Health Organization (WHO)
Avenue Appia
1211 Geneva 27
Switzerland

World Hospitals
126 Albert Street
London NW1 7NF
U.K.

World Neighbours
5116 North Portland Avenue
Oklahoma City
Oklahoma 73112
U.S.A.

Yale University School of Medicine
333 Cedar Street
New Haven
Connecticut 06510
U.S.A.

Space for your own notes and contacts

Space for your own notes and contacts

Space for your own notes and contacts

Space for your own notes and contacts

Space for your own notes and contacts

Space for your own notes and contacts

Space for your own notes and contacts

Space for your own notes and contacts

Space for your own notes and contacts

Space for your own notes and contacts

Space for your own notes and contacts

Space for your own notes and contacts

www.ingramcontent.com/pod-product-compliance
Lightning Source LLC
Chambersburg PA
CBHW060044030426
42334CB00019B/2478